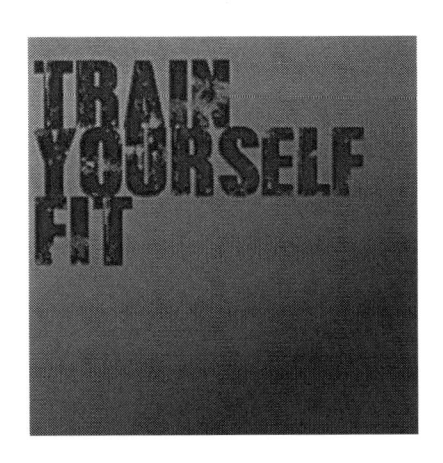

www.trainyourselffit.com

Bodyweight Exercise

10 principles that will get you the results *you* want from *your* training

Copyright © 2017 Ben Herd

This book is copyright under the Berne Convention.

No reproduction without permission.

All rights reserved.

The right of Ben Herd to be identified as the author of this work has been asserted in accordance with sections 77 and 78 of the Copyright, Designs and Patents Act, 1988.

A catalogue record for this book is available from the British Library

ISBN: 978-0-9933938-2-2

Published and illustrated by Ben Herd

Printed by CreateSpace, an Amazon.com Company

Disclaimer

The author and publisher of this material is in no manner whatsoever responsible for any injury that may occur through following the instructions in this material. The activities, physical and otherwise, described herein are described for informational purposes only, and the reader should always consult a physician before engaging in any of them.

To all trainers, no matter your level – liberate yourselves through knowledge so you can go forth doing what you know is absolutely right for *you* and *you alone*

A massive thank you to everyone that read this book before it was published – you know who you are

'Being wise doesn't mean to "add" more, being wise means to be able to get off sophistication and be simply simple.'

Bruce Lee

(from *Jeet kune do: Bruce Lee's Commentaries on the Martial Way*)

About the Author

Ben Herd lives in South West Devon close to Dartmoor National Park. He holds a Level 3 Certificate in Personal Training and an Honours Degree in the Arts including a qualification in Sport, Fitness and Management. His interests include writing, drawing and illustration, physical fitness and martial arts. As well as the *Bodyweight Exercise* series of books, he is also the author of the novel *Jungle of Gold*, and runs www.trainyourselffit.com.

Also by this author (Fiction):

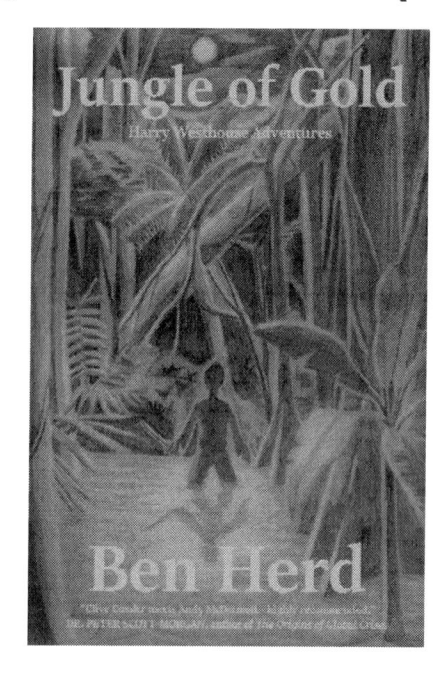

When Harry Westhouse and his friends went in search of a place and a treasure lost to history on what they believed would be the adventure of their lives, he never for a moment thought that they would end up fighting just to stay alive . . .

Ever since he was a small boy and his father told him a story about sighting ruins amongst the remote jungle of Burma whilst fighting there during World War II, Harry has dreamed of finding the place whose very existence was curiously denied by the indigenous population.

Now an archaeologist against his father's wishes, Harry's research has led him to believe that the place his father saw could not only rewrite the history books of Burma, but could yield rich rewards for him and his friends that no one else even suspects exist.

But the risks are high. Harry knows Burma is a country off limits to outsiders and that the Indian-Burmese border they must cross to reach their destination is a potential war zone. If they are to succeed, they must remain unseen, hidden in the jungle.

Yet the jungle is not as deserted as they had hoped. Very quickly disturbing occurrences show them that they are not alone, and events see them separated and running for their lives as they become witnesses to murder. Meeting a foe they could never have anticipated, they must fight for each other to survive as the past and the present collide to make them pay for what they have found.

"Brilliant story, can't wait for more from this author." IAN HAMBLY-BROOKS, Amazon review

"Thrilling book, full of suspense and kept me on my toes right till the end. Highly recommended!"
YIKAI ZHANG, proprietor of *ManimalZYK*

"Kept me hooked from start to finish and loved the many plot twists throughout. Very exciting storyline."
CHRIS RICHARDS, Amazon review

Table of Contents

Introduction: Why I have decided to write these books	i-iv
Why bodyweight exercises only?	1
Some necessary information	5
Principle 1: Set Goals: Using the SMART approach	9
Principle 2: Simplicity is Key: Do fewer exercises better	17
Principle 3: Consistent Frequency	29
Principle 4: Progressive Overload	41
Principle 5: Correct Form: Focus upon this before anything else	47
Principle 6: Mental Focus: Using the mind to improve your results	51
Principle 7: Patience: Learn to listen to your body	57
Principle 8: Periodisation: Balancing exercise with rest and recovery	61
Principle 9: Different Approaches: Eke out every gain from each exercise	65
Principle 10: The Importance of Strength: Train specifically for strength from time to time to gain more size	71
Conclusion	75
References	76
Appendix 1: Why building max strength will also help to build endurance	77

Introduction: Why I have decided to write these books

Health and fitness: a simple phrase describing something that should be simple in execution to achieve and maintain. But there is a problem.

The fitness community, whether experienced online, or in person, can be a very confusing place. Nearly everyone seems to have a different opinion regarding what works or what does not to achieve the best results regarding any number of things, whether this relates to what exercises to perform or even a specific way to perform any given exercise.

Similarly, nutrition can easily be mistaken for a minefield, fraught as this subject is with varieties of diet too many to count.

Both of these problems can be quickly encountered by simply doing a quick search on YouTube, for example. This will quickly reveal a number of different approaches to the same exercise topic. And this begs the question of anyone willing to use their own decision making skills of analysis applied to what they are watching—rather than just going along with it because the experts or the maker of the video says so—to ask:

'So, what actually works best?'

Or, 'Who should I believe?'

Then there's the whole problem of how strong a frightening number of people appear to be on YouTube. YouTube seems to be filled with self-made gymnasts or powerlifters, performing feats of strength most of us can only dream of, or at least currently believe we will never be able to perform.

Disheartening? It can be. Or, as I prefer to approach this problem, inspirational. After all, we are all human. We all have the same basic attributes gifted to us from birth, so why, if these people can do these things, shouldn't everyone be able to? Everybody is capable of fantastic things. Provided you put your mind to it and allot the suitable amount of hard work and dedication to your efforts, anything is achievable.

However, there is also another problem that the presence of all these experts raises. This is the main one that I intend to address in this book in as simple but as effective a manner as possible: the distraction caused by information overload.

It is certainly a good thing that so many people are willing to share what they know. But all too often what is being shared are just different programs or personal opinions, causing people to constantly skip from one workout to another in an elusive search for the one that will someday give them the results they desire.

This, to me, seems like a fundamentally wrong approach. Just acting on anything out of blind faith, or misinformation, is going to fail.

Success comes from true understanding of why you are doing something, and in the case of exercise, I believe this means that everyone needs an understanding of the fundamental rules or principles that will make any form of exercise or workout program work. More importantly, it helps to know why you are doing something a particular way so that you can stick to it with conviction. This is what I will give you in this book.

But what qualifies me to do this, you might ask?

Well, I believe I have a very useful perspective from which to approach the problem facing all of us, myself included, of how to develop the necessary strength to get to these perhaps seemingly unreachable levels of strength. I am a qualified personal trainer too, but even more important than that, I believe, is personal experience. In this regard, I believe that I have a useful insight that many trainers don't have into the hurdles many people—especially those that have never been exercise fanatics or gym bunnies—face in getting strong and fit, or indeed even where to start. So this book can be used by those both new to, or more experienced in exercise, to stop both groups making unnecessary mistakes due to information overload.

Essentially, I have always been into 'keeping fit', as many people would say, since my early teens. There is a wonderful saying that when we are young, we are made from rubber and magic. In other words, we can recover from anything, and get away with doing many exercises with bad form, but still get results and avoid, or at least overcome injuries in a hurry. Consequently, I was pretty quickly doing exercises like assisted one-armed pull-ups, handstand push-ups, dragon flags and weighted dips, and, I know now, without having followed sensible progressions that would have made me so much stronger whilst achieving these exercises in a much safer and effective manner. And importantly, with fewer injuries.

Then though, about five years ago now, a kind lady decided to shunt my car. This resulted in a whiplash injury that, as it turned out, would pretty much destroy my back muscles. Everything went stiff, achy and weak, and remained so for months. I went from doing easy sets of forty five to fifty push-ups to not being able to perform a single full push-up, since I just couldn't hold the plank position in which push-ups are done any more.

Adding bad news to what already seemed a bad enough situation, I then developed epilepsy. Anyone who has seen someone having a seizure will know that you literally try to curl yourself in half the wrong way, so that your spine hyperextends alarmingly and your head tries to disappear behind you. Consequently, any damage the whiplash had caused to my back was badly exacerbated.

This was followed with a year of medically advised inactivity because doctors were clueless to the cause of my epilepsy and so wanted to eliminate too much exercise as a factor. The result for me was a consequential gain in weight, mostly around the midriff, since the medication I was on literally made me ravenous. Indeed, I fell into a 'see food and eat it diet,' and of course my fitness suffered as a result. In the process though, I think I gained a very useful insight into what many people face when deciding to get fit from a position of being far from ideally mobile and overweight, as well as what causes people to get to this place in the first place.

As a result, learning to start all over again became key to me. Nothing was easy anymore. I just had to be humble and start from scratch. For example, I had to start to learn push-ups all over again by doing them stood up, against a wall. So I had been reduced to doing the most basic version of an exercise that I had thought was basic before when done in its full version on the floor. Yet the floor version was now something completely unattainable for me. Indeed, even push-ups against a wall seemed fairly challenging. Something that was also true of virtually all of the other exercises I had previously been so strong in.

Subsequently, I quickly learned through personal trial and error, and hours of educating myself, just how to get strong again, or at least stronger. This time around though, I was using a much more informed approach, since I had to contend with all my weaknesses, instead of just jumping in straight away with the hard exercises that had seemed so easy before. I had no choice.

Taking a positive from a negative then, what I gained, I believe, is a great amount of knowledge. Knowledge I would now like to share, to show anyone, particularly beginners starting from scratch like I had to, that you can absolutely achieve exactly what you want in strength terms so long as you have the right approach. Any goal can be achieved, so long as you apply the step-by-step approach and principles I present in this book. With this information, you can build upon seemingly small, insignificant steps until in time, you will be able to perform exercises that you might never have dreamed of.

Sure, this information is hardly revolutionary and is certain to be out there already on the internet or in libraries all over the world, but in a widely disseminated and disconnected fashion. So my goal in this series of books is to cut straight to the point and collect the fundamental information that matters together in one place, and in a linked way. This way, you will always have a useful reference tool to save yourself time researching these things. Time that can instead be better spent on achieving the fitness goals you seek.

What I present here in this first book then is a set of 10 principles that can be applied to any and all workouts to give you success. They are as key to your exercise success as the foundations are to the structure of a house, or the letters of an alphabet are to a written language. They will be the building blocks for your success. So these principles should be learnt first before proceeding onto the other books in this series where I will deal with subjects like detailed analysis of individual exercises and subjects like programming your workouts. This way, you can start to apply the knowledge you gain from this book to the actual process of exercise right from the outset as you go forwards, to gain as much experience in terms of physically applying this knowledge as possible.

Since these principles are so fundamental, you should also be able to take something away from this book, and indeed the others, regardless of your current level in terms of exercise experience or fitness. By the end of this book you should see how to exercise for success in terms of gaining the best results from any exercise program you may already be doing. You should see that getting results from your exercise really shouldn't be that complicated to achieve, but that all you need is to apply a little time and consistent effort to make yourself fitter and stronger for life.

I hope you enjoy the journey, and learn to enjoy living in the body you were gifted with if you don't already.

Why bodyweight exercises only?

There is no need to complicate this answer. Purely and simply, the use of bodyweight as opposed to weights is convenient for the following reasons:

Functionality/day-to-day carryover:

Every day we move our bodies around all day long. Therefore if we learn to move this fixed weight around in more challenging positions than our daily lives demand, our daily lives will be so much easier. This is essentially a bodyweight equivalent of how the Romans used to train their soldiers with training swords and shields made deliberately heavier than the real weapons. As a result, when using the real thing, the sword and shield would have seemed much easier to use by comparison, and could be used much faster and for longer.

Bodyweight exercises also require moving our entire bodies through space in various challenging positions. This means they will develop a high level of coordination as you learn to contract lots of muscles throughout your body in a simultaneous effort so that you learn to feel your body working as a single, unified entity. This is how we naturally use our bodies day-to-day, for everyday motions like walking or getting out of a car. Many weighted exercises do this too, but this is just a default mode with almost all bodyweight exercises, guaranteeing this will be a feature of you training.

In essence then, bodyweight exercises will heighten body awareness. This is an essential quality to develop when progressing in any exercises to gain the maximum results (as you will read under Principle 5) by learning to do all exercises absolutely correctly.

Safety:

This links in with the above point. Since you move your bodyweight around all day, it is both more practical and often far safer to exercise with just your bodyweight utilised as the load than it is to go into a gym and load up a barbell with a heavy weight. This is because too many people fall prey to letting their egos take over where weights are concerned. And a heavy weight, if disrespected, can easily and quickly cause harm.

By comparison, because of the nature of the way that bodyweight exercises are scalable by the version of the exercise you do, it is easy to alter the difficulty of bodyweight exercises even though the load—your bodyweight—remains exactly the same throughout.

So, if you try a full push-up from the top position (though you should always start from lying on the floor), the worst that can happen is you fall to the floor if you fail the rep, or you can just put your knees down. But at no point are you going to be crushed by a heavy barbell. Similarly, in a full dip, you will only be able to go as deep as you can, which, however deep that may be, you can just drop off the bars if required and so end the rep there.

Cost effectiveness:

At the time of writing, to purchase weights, it will cost you about £1 in British currency for every pound of weight that you purchase. Needless to say then, buying weights gets costly in a hurry, not to mention all of the other equipment like benches that you might not have room to store or house anyway.

Yes, it is true that with bodyweight exercise, to get the best results you will still require certain basic equipment like parallel bars, a pull-up bar and perhaps even gymnastic rings. But this is all still cheap in comparison to weights, with all of this equipment costing around £60 - £80 in total if you shop around.

Enjoyment/achievement:

This one may be a little bit biased in terms of personal preference on my part. But generally speaking, if you move into learning exercises like one arm push-ups and handstands, or indeed just many of the more fundamental exercises like push-ups, there is a sense of body mastery and achievement that you just don't get from using weights alone. To do a handstand, for example, you have to control your whole body from your fingers to your toes, and the feeling of achievement when you start to actually control the balance in such a movement is beyond compare of anything I ever garnered from just lifting weights.

Convenience:

Time is one of the main reasons people give as an excuse not to exercise, so cut out the time required to get to the gym (not to mention the cost of gym memberships) and use this commute time more effectively to workout at home. Also, there is the space issue mentioned under cost effectiveness above. The Chinese have a saying that you can practice Kung Fu in the space a tiger can lie down in, and whilst you won't need to be housing any tigers any time soon, a bit of floor space will get you a long way for a whole plethora of bodyweight exercises. Space anyone should be able to find.

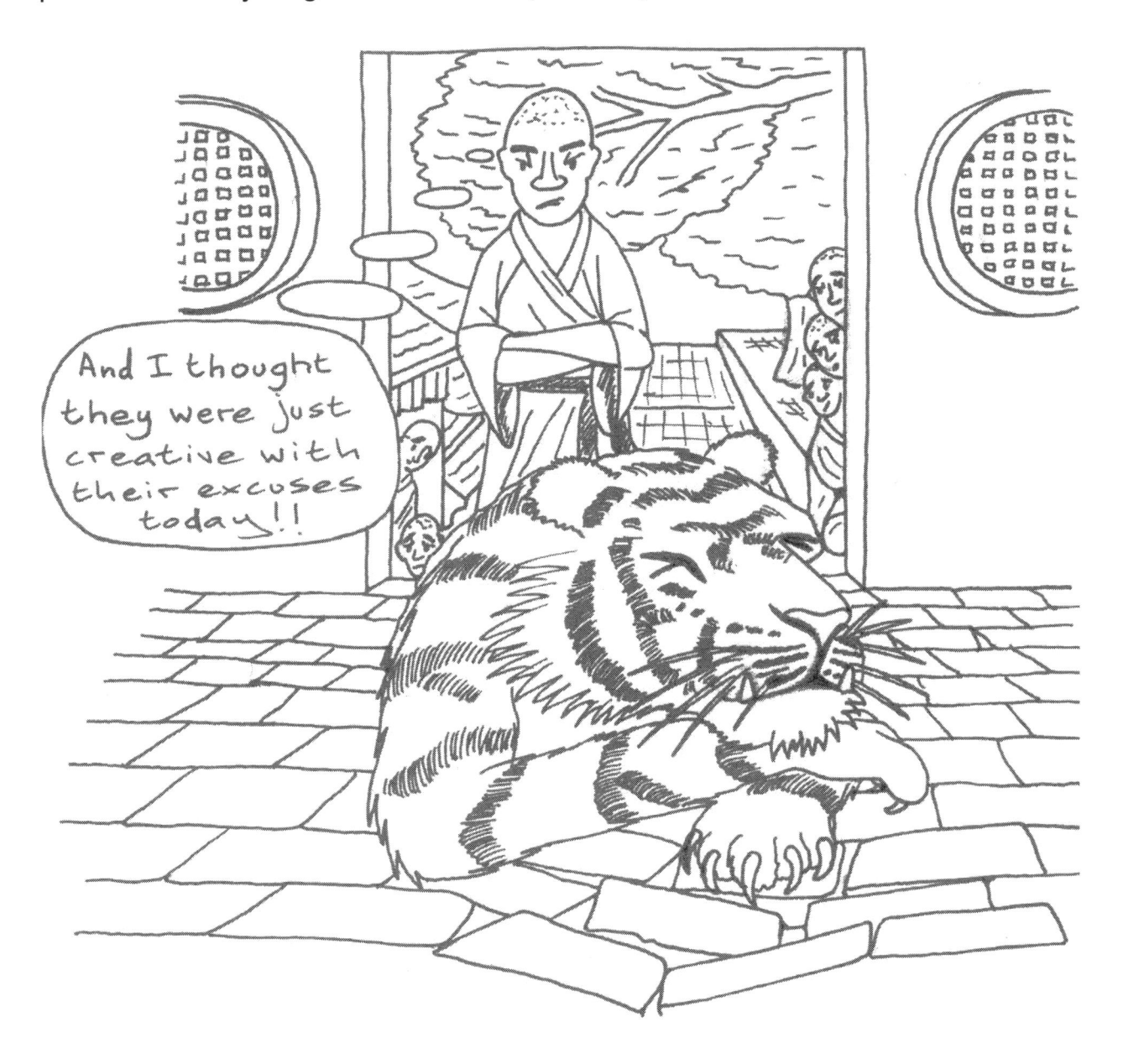

What it all adds up to:

In conclusion then, utilising bodyweight exercises for your training will remove the most common excuses that people come up with when trying to avoid exercising, simply because using bodyweight as the resistance for your workouts removes so many obstacles to exercise. So press on and get the results you want, excuse free.

Some necessary information

To best understand the principles highlighted in this book, it will simplify the process to first give you some brief but necessary information relating to how resistance exercise works.

Resistance workouts are directed towards developing strength and in connection with this, muscle mass.

So it is important to understand that there are two kinds or categories of strength that you can develop:

1. *Maximum strength*, or what can also be regarded as brute strength
2. *Strength endurance*, which is the ability to perform strength movements for an extended period of time

How much strength you use or more precisely the level of effort and percentage of the working muscles you use during a workout is called the *intensity* level. This really relates to the percentage of your total potential effort applied to each movement.

If you were to perform a single repetition (rep) lifting the heaviest weight you are capable of lifting, you would have performed a lift with your 1 rep max weight (1 RM).

So intensity is usually expressed as a percentage of your 1 RM weight. The higher the intensity at which you work, but for lower reps, the more maximum strength you would be using and so working to develop. (Though the level of effort applied is also affected by other factors to be explained later, like good form and mental focus).

If however you reduce the weight you use, to perform more reps, or with bodyweight exercises perform a version of an exercise that allows you to perform a higher number of repetitions, the lower the intensity of the exercise will be. Concurrently though, your muscles will be able to lift this weight for longer. So a lower load with more reps will work muscular endurance more, developing your muscles to work for a more prolonged period of time, which is also a very important strength attribute in terms of general conditioning. After all, we are more often called upon to go for long periods in life than to lift heavy objects.

Since building muscle mass results best from working elements of both of these types of strength however, and of course functionality in the real world does too, building higher levels of maximum strength will be the single element of strength that will have the best carry over initially to both areas of your strength training. This maximum strength will form the foundation on which strength endurance can then be built with heavier loads since you can start moving back into the hypertrophy (muscle building) rep ranges in your sets (see Principle 10).

In other words, the steps in the process towards building muscle are important.

1. First, build higher levels of maximum strength with low reps to increase the loads you can lift in total, focusing on this at least some of the time
2. Then you can start to work on being able to handle these higher loads for a longer duration again by starting to add more reps to your sets

The main point I want you to take away for the moment then is that building high levels of maximum strength is an important prerequisite. This applies both in terms of functionality, through improving your overall conditioning (endurance), and in terms of muscle growth. (For more detail about how resistance workouts can benefit muscular endurance and the cardiovascular system, see Appendix 1 at the end of this book).

To better visualise why building maximum strength is beneficial to muscular endurance, consider this. Whilst initially you may have to do fewer reps with a heavier weight, as you progress, you will be able to lift that weight for more reps, and have obviously developed the ability to lift a heavier weight. Even if you have to decrease the load a little at first to start increasing your rep ranges again however, and build this up over time, by having increased your max strength, this reduced load will still nevertheless be a percentage of a heavier load than you could have lifted before since it will be a percentage of a heavier load to start with

(i.e. 60 % of 200 pounds, which may be your example 1 RM weight, would be more than 60 % of 180 pounds if that was your 1 RM weight.)

So at least some of the time in your training, even if your main goal is to build ascetically pleasing muscle more than getting really strong and functionally fit, you should focus on training your maximum strength to maximise your muscular growth in the most efficient way (see also Principle 10 for more detail).

Also, if you are struggling to increase your maximal number of reps at an exercise like pull-ups, focusing on developing your maximal strength in place of rep numbers will help to get you over the plateau (as shown by using the method of different approaches that again focus on muscular tension over reps: see Principle 9). A higher level of maximal strength will again allow you to perform more reps more easily. All of which will be explained in much more detail within the principles in this book.

Principle 1
Set Goals

Using the SMART approach

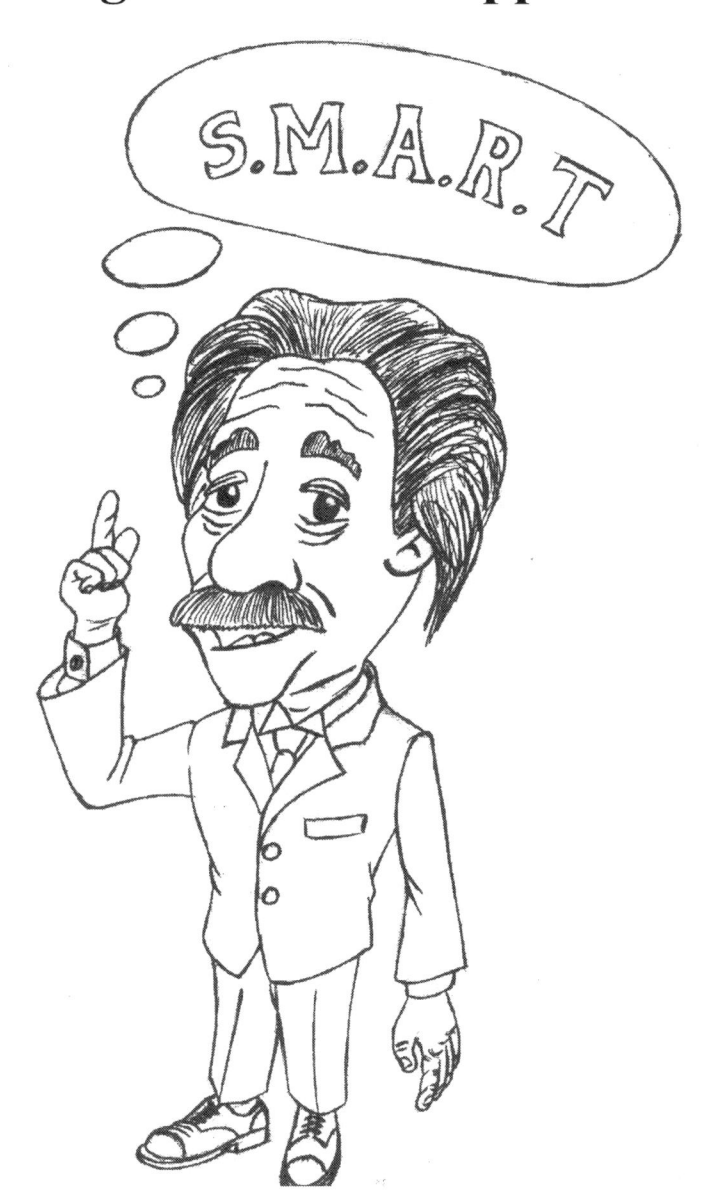

"Imagination is everything. It is the preview of life's coming attractions."
Albert Einstein

To achieve anything in life, you need to know exactly what it is you want to achieve. In a word, you need a *plan*. Something to work towards. This is why the first thing you should do before embarking on any kind of exercise program is to sit down and take time to set yourself goals so that you know *exactly* what you are going to be working to achieve. Even if you are a regular exerciser already, ask yourself if you have ever done/do this, and if not, start to implement this into your training and watch the results come.

Setting yourself goals is a simple process, made more so by the application of a SMART approach. SMART is an acronym for the following:

- Specificity
- Measurable
- Achievable/Attainable
- Realistic/Relevant
- Time-bound

Here is what each of these five points relate to, and why they will ensure you start to get results from whatever exercise program you choose to do, resistance based or otherwise.

Specificity

Whatever training you are doing, it must be specifically directed towards achieving the results or goals that *you* want to get from *your* exercise. You must be very certain to specify the exact criteria of what you want to achieve, which will allow you to focus on your goals, and *only* your goals in your training.

For example, if you want your legs to grow, you must work your legs directly with the relevant exercises. You would not work your upper body to achieve this leg-specific goal, and you would not do exercises designed to build endurance in your leg muscles if you want to build muscular size. (This is where knowledge of different training approaches is useful. I touch upon this briefly in Principle 10 of this book so you know what approaches produce what results). Or if you want to lose weight, you must ensure that your diet specifically targets this, by dropping the number of calories you eat on a daily basis, whilst incorporating the correct sorts of fat burning exercise into your exercise regimen.

Identifying your specific goals, then, will make you work in a very targeted way towards the overall outcome that you are seeking to achieve, rather than just following some vague, general program. This is key, both physically and mentally, because it is all too easy to become distracted by the latest fad in exercise, especially if you work out in a gym, or read a lot on the subject. But identifying your specific needs will provide you with the necessary mental focus to stick to *your own* program to achieve the results *you* desire from your training.

The simplest way to make your training specific is to ask the following question:

Is this particular exercise going to help me achieve the results/goals I am seeking?

If it is not, don't do this exercise and replace it with one that does target what you want to achieve. Otherwise you will just be watering down your results by wasting time and energy that could be better applied towards achieving your specific goal.

This remains true even if specificity means you end up doing fewer exercises overall (hard to believe for many, but Principle 2 explains why fewer exercises will give better results.)

So identify exactly what it is you want to achieve, which moves us onto the next points.

Measurable

There must be some way to measure the results from what you are doing. Otherwise, you will not know if what you are doing is effective or not.

Some examples of measuring your results are:

- To weigh yourself regularly, at a set time and on a set day each week, to ensure that you are measuring this in a scientific and accurate way
- Using a tape measure to regularly measure your various body areas, such as at the end of each exercise cycle or period of say four to six weeks (an exercise cycle/period is just the length of time that you stick

to your regular pattern of working out before taking a longer period of rest, such as a total rest week)
- Taking before and after photos for each period of training, taken in the same place and with the same lighting
- Going to a leisure centre to use a body composition machine that will tell you how your fat percentage is changing
- Recording your exercise in an exercise log so you can note when exercises are starting to feel easier, when your form is improving, or indeed when things are still feeling hard

Measuring your progress then is an absolutely essential thing to do, and will require you to record your results. I would recommend a simple notebook to record your measurements, but any method by which you want to record these is fine. Just so long as you do so in some regard. Only through keeping a record can you compare your results over time and so assess if you are getting the results you want, when you want. As seemingly simple as this is, it is also the best way to keep yourself motivated; by seeing what you are achieving, you will be spurred on to keep going.

Similarly, you must record everything that you do in terms of exercise in each workout, so that you can look back and see what exercises or approaches worked, or perhaps what didn't, to help your future progress by allowing you to refine and adapt your workouts as necessary. Keep your records simple, like recording:

- The exercise and variant of that exercise that you did
- The number of reps and sets you did
- How long you rested for between sets
- How much weight you used if you added weight to a bodyweight movement
- A few brief notes on things like how the exercise felt—whether easy or hard—and how your form was or where it can be improved next time. This will improve your focus in your subsequent workouts

When you review your exercise progress then, like at the end of an exercise cycle, these records will show you what worked or indeed what you did that failed to get you results. But be honest with yourself in this process, since you will only cheat yourself otherwise.

For example, if you skipped workouts and recorded as much, you will see that this, and not the program itself was the problem when you come to review your progress. Otherwise, you may forget or deny to yourself that you did this and so blame the program. Such an oversight will potentially cause you to fall into the trap of constantly switching exercise programs, and this will only doom you to failure (for reasons explained in Principle 2).

If you find that you are regularly missing your goals, it may also be very helpful to start adding number values to your goals, so that you push yourself hard enough to actually get the results you are seeking. This links back to being specific, since you can specify things like losing a set amount of weight by a set time, to keep your progress on track if you are someone that finds it hard to push yourself hard enough in your workouts for whatever reason. This way, when you are in the midst of a rep that seems too hard, you can visualise your goal(s), and get the extra spur of motivation you need to keep driving towards those goals.

Achievable/Attainable

Quite simply, the goals you specify for yourself must be set at a level so that you can actually achieve them.

This doesn't mean that the goals you set must be restricted. Just that you need to acknowledge that to achieve anything from your exercise, it will take time, and you need to break your goals into manageable, achievable chunks by dividing them into the following:

- Short term goals
- Medium term goals
- Long term goals

This also relates to the time-bound section of SMART, but where achievable/attainable is concerned, you need to realise that if you set your sights too high, too soon, you only set yourself up for disappointment. By failing to hit a goal set too high, you will only dishearten yourself and so decrease your own motivation, especially if you are someone that struggles to remain motivated.

So instead, work clever, and realise that small steps, i.e. seemingly limited short term goals, build into bigger, more impressive intermediate steps (medium term goals). In this manner, small and intermediate goals will accumulate and lead you to your ultimate goals—your long term goals.

Realistic/Relevant

This ties in with the above. As stated, you need to be realistic with yourself in terms of what you can achieve, and so set goals relevant to your level and what you are aiming to achieve in terms of fitness. Don't worry about what anyone else is doing. You need to drop your ego and ensure that *you* are working at the correct level for yourself at all times. As the old gym saying goes: 'Leave your ego outside of the door.'

Also, acknowledge immediately that only *you* know what *you* are personally capable of, so that you will accept that this process of setting your goals will take a little bit of time to finesse.

In itself, setting goals is a learning process since you will learn about yourself and your capabilities. This means it will initially take a little bit of fine tuning to learn what goals are realistic to you. But don't be disheartened by this; just accept it for what it is: a learning curve.

Most especially then, realise that what you can achieve and so what is realistic for you at any given time relates directly to your current level of conditioning. So keep your goals, especially your short term goals, relevant to the level at which you presently sit to ensure you can hit your goals.

Time-bound

Going back to the short, medium and long term goal model, time-bound simply means that you need to add a time period to each of these goal stages. So you may set four weeks as the time in which to achieve your short term goals, eight weeks from your start point in which to achieve your medium term goals, and twelve weeks from the start point as the time in which you aim to achieve your long term goal.

Whatever the time period you add though, remember the other points above, particularly the need to be realistic.

Summary

So, there you have it, a very simple but highly effective way to ensure that you effectively organise your workouts in order to get the best results, and, more importantly, the results that *you alone* actually want. There really is no need to work to some vague, overriding goal like 'to get fitter,' that is little use to anyone. Or, indeed, to follow someone else's program, such as that of a certain celebrity.

Also, as a parting thought relating to goals, don't set your goals too high with regards to always working towards too many different goals. Two to three goals for each stage of your training should be plenty to create real focus and so the drive to succeed. Plus this will massively increase the odds of you actually reaching your goals.

In brief, your checklist is as follows:

- Make sure the exercises you do are actually specific to what it is that you are aiming to achieve so none of your precious time and effort is being wasted
- Make sure you can measure your progress in some way so that you can actually monitor the changes occurring to your body. To do this, always record what you are doing to remove any uncertainty from the process
- Make sure your goals can actually be achieved so you are not setting yourself up for potential disappointment and so failure by making yourself despondent when you don't get the results you were hoping to see. Remember, so long as you record everything, you can assess why you may have failed and so learn how to work smarter to achieve your goals next time. This will also prevent you demotivating yourself if it was just your approach that was wrong in some way, like perhaps having set yourself an unrealistic time in which to achieve your goals. After all, we learn best from our mistakes
- Acknowledge that progress takes time so you can be realistic in your expectations, to ensure that you are working at a level relevant to your current capabilities
- Set time limits on all your goals, short, medium and long term to keep yourself motivated and on track to success
- Limit your total number of goals for maximum focus and success

Principle 2
Simplicity is Key

Do fewer exercises better

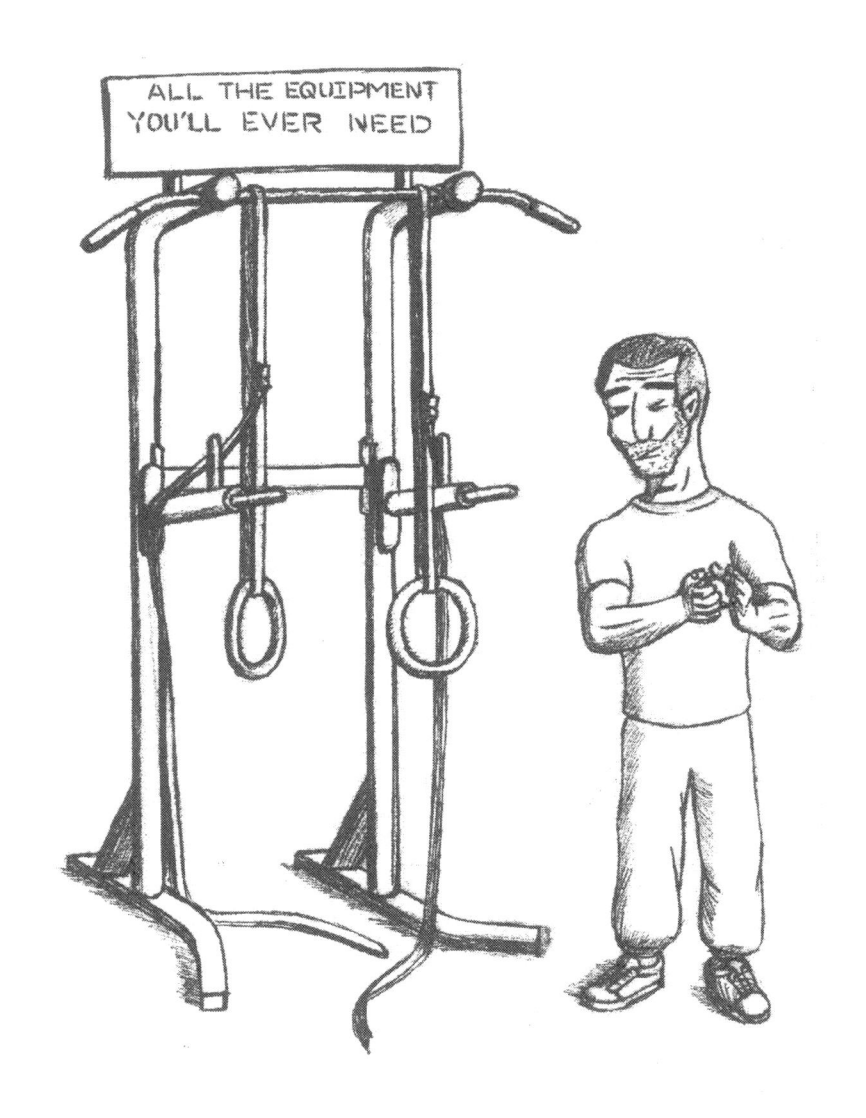

"Do nothing that is of no use." Miyamoto Musashi

If you look at someone who is a master of anything, they have a way of making what they do seem so easy. Whether it is the seemingly effortless way in which an athlete moves, or the way in which a good teacher can break down a complex process into easier to digest steps that we can understand. In essence then, these 'masters' have simplified what they do, but gained the maximum results and benefits from doing so.

Think about this for a moment though, and you'll quickly realise this is a logical outcome. They have, after all, focused upon doing fewer things, but in a better way. They have *specialised*, so that they don't do anything that is not essential to success in whatever their chosen endeavour. As a result, they have gained far more practice at the thing upon which they have focused their attentions, and thus reached a level of mastery that is beyond most ordinary people who split their attentions and efforts between many things. This is why a street fighter who has mastered a few techniques will always beat a martial artist who has had to practice hundreds of different techniques. After all, the old axiom is that practice makes perfect, and practicing fewer things means more practice time, and so a higher level of accomplishment.

What this points to is that a diffusion of effort is often a bad thing. That complexity can and will dilute results. So, where an exercise program is concerned, simplicity is likewise the best way to go.

By simplicity, I mean restricting your efforts to doing only what is necessary to get the results you desire. This may involve doing a fair number of different things since fitness targets so many different areas of performance, with a definition of physical fitness including:

- Muscular strength
- Muscular endurance
- Cardiovascular fitness
- Flexibility
- Motor skills: attributes like coordination, balance and speed

Nevertheless, we can still simplify the things we do, and so gain the maximum results from these things, whilst always operating upon the idea that *less is definitely more*. (The very reason why it is easier to get more success by restricting the number of goals we work towards).

More especially, we can do **fewer exercises, better.**

This may seem anathema to many who like to hit each individual muscle or muscle group with several different exercises, as a bodybuilder might. This is not to say they are doing anything wrong, as bodybuilders have the express aim of developing each muscle to its ascetic best. That is their *specific* goal.

But in terms of developing an all-around, aesthetically pleasing physique with healthy levels of muscle and a healthy fat percentage, and one that is capable of high levels of functional strength, for people who don't have hours to spend in the gym and eating tonnes of protein, doing fewer exercises better can still give you fantastic results. Furthermore, you can still gain very high levels of strength with this approach.

Why does doing fewer exercises performed better work?

In a word, because it guarantees **consistency.** And where exercise is concerned, consistency is key for the following reason.

The body has to go through two steps in order for you to gain strength, and muscle mass. These two steps are:

1. Neurological adaptations (adaptations related to the nervous system)
2. Muscular hypertrophy (muscular growth)

These two steps have to occur in this order. In other words, until your nervous system has made adaptations to the new workload, such as a new exercise that you subject your body to, you will not be able to grow larger muscles very effectively.

Neurological Adaptations and the Strength Development Process

What exactly does this mean?

Neurological just relates to our nervous system.

The nervous system is like a complex of telephone wires that relay messages all over our bodies, composed of a few key components:

- The central nervous system (CNS), which consists of the brain and spinal cord

- The peripheral nervous system (PNS), which consists of sensory neurons (nerves) and motor neurons. Information from our sense organs, like the eyes, ears, and sense receptors under our skin is passed back to the CNS via sensory nerves. This is so that a relevant response can be decided upon. This response is then made to happen by messages being sent from our CNS to places like our muscles along the motor nerves so that the required action is carried out by our bodies

To explain the two adaptations that occur in relation to exercise, it is only necessary to speak of the brain and the motor nerves.

For a muscle to contract to cause any desired movement, messages must pass from the brain (CNS) to the muscle in question. These messages are transmitted to the muscle by motor neurons (neuron just means nerve).

In keeping with the analogy of the nervous system being like a complex of telephone wires, a motor nerve is like a large mains telephone cable. When this large cable reaches the muscle it controls, it branches out into lots of smaller wires, like those branching off a main telephone pylon into individual houses upon reaching a housing estate.

In a muscle though, the houses represent individual muscle fibres. Depending on the type of muscle fibres within that muscle (slow or fast twitch), the size of the main cable of the motor nerve is either smaller or larger respectively. The smaller slow twitch fibre motor nerves also only branch out to around 100 muscle fibres, compared to around 10,000 muscle fibres in the case of the larger, fast twitch motor nerves.

Back to the phone analogy then. When a motor neuron passes the phone call to each of the homes (muscle fibres) it speaks to and so controls, all of the phones receive the message. So 100% of the muscle fibres are activated by the message. None of the individual fibres or phones can be activated separate from the whole, and so this is called the 'all or none' principle.

Because the motor nerve and the muscle fibres it talks to, or activates, are as such an inseparable whole, this whole is called a motor unit.

In terms of the nervous system, efficiency relates to the frequency at which these messages pass along the motor nerves, and also to how well the message is received on the other end, at the muscle. So again, using the phone analogy, this can be compared to the strength of the reception where the phone calls (nerve messages, or impulses) are received.

How well the message is received at the muscle end of the motor unit is dependent on how many motor units, and so how many smaller wires to the individual houses (muscle fibres), are activated to receive the messages. The more motor units that receive the message, the greater the reception.

Consequently, how many of these muscle fibres receive the message to contract relates directly to the percentage of a muscle that you are able to contract to perform a given action. A percentage that can only be increased by improving upon how many motor units can be recruited to speak to a muscle to make it perform the action being asked of it.

So think of learning to recruit more motor units as laying more mains phone lines. The more mains lines you can lay down, the more individual lines can disperse out from these mains lines into the muscle at the other end.

The more mains lines you can recruit to send messages, the greater the strength of a muscular contraction can be then since you can talk to more muscle fibres within the muscle in question and so contract the greatest possible percentage of the muscle in question. As this percentage rises, so your strength increases. In untrained individuals, around 30% of the muscle's total fibres can be activated, but as you train and improve upon this, around 50% of your total muscle fibres can be taught to contract.

MORE MOTOR NERVES = MORE MOTOR UNITS

MORE MOTOR UNITS = MORE STRENGTH

Other Important Neurological Adaptations for Strength Development

Initially then, as you start to do a new exercise, your brain has to learn how to talk to your muscles more effectively. Consequently, you cannot tense your muscle very hard, so that you are using your existing muscle mass inefficiently. (Remember, only about 30% of your muscles' total fibres can be contracted before training). But the more you perform a given exercise, the more motor units you learn to recruit to help perform the action.

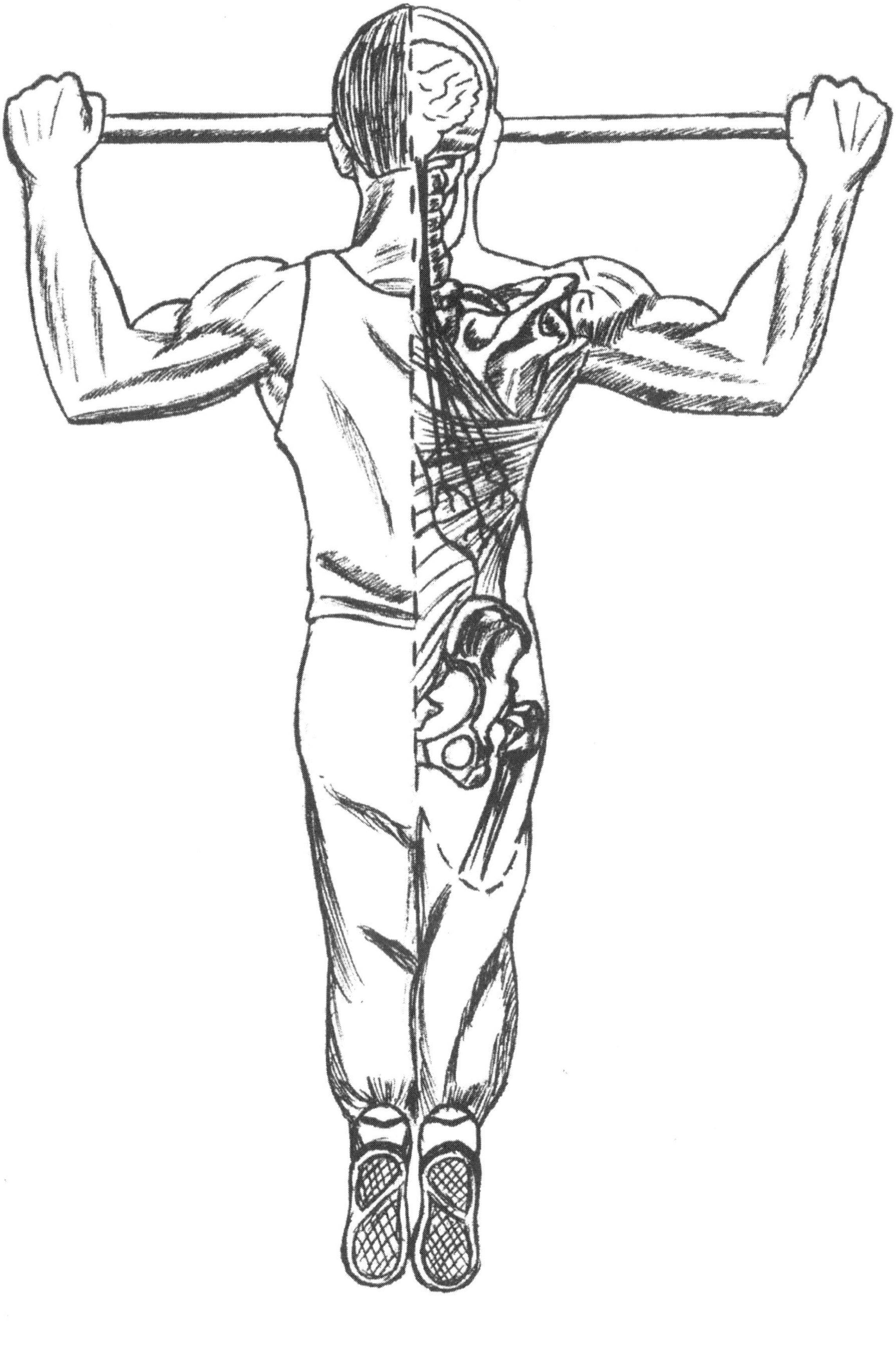

Another neurological adaptation your exercise will cause is to improve the frequency with which the nerve impulses (messages) travel down the motor units. This is like upgrading your dial-up internet connection to a fibre-optic network, and will further strengthen your muscular contractions since your muscle is told to contract more often in the same amount of time, increasing the phone reception at your muscle, if you like. This is because the frequency of a nerve impulse is what tells your muscles how hard they are being asked to contract.

GREATER FREQUENCY OF IMPULSES = HARDER CONTRACTION

Think of how these adaptations will help you in your everyday life then. For example, if you walk up a steep hill, but, for the sake of illustration, only have two motor neurons telling your muscles to contract, you will be working twice as hard as someone that has taught four motor neurons to talk to the same muscles. This is because those two neurons will have to be carrying all of the workload, so they will be doing 100% of the work compared to 50% of the work in the person with four motor neurons, and you can only get half as many messages to your muscles in the same amount of time. So their nerves are doing half the work that yours are. Not forgetting that you will also be using a lower percentage of your muscle mass as a result, so that the same effort is also twice as intense for you since your level of strength is already lower to start with.

Muscles are also powered by your cardiovascular system, since muscle cells are a site of respiration—a process that requires the efforts of the cardiovascular system to provide the products required for this—which means that the person with twice as many motor neurons will have better muscular endurance. This is because they can call upon a greater percentage of their muscle fibres—and by extension muscle cells—to perform the same task, which is of course spreading the workload. So the same effort you are partaking in, i.e. walking up the hill, is easier for them. This is why building strength is the precursor for improving other physical attributes like muscular endurance. Unlocking more strength via neurological adaptations also unlocks cardiovascular system adaptations relating to endurance, like better oxygen absorption at the site of your muscles (see also Appendix 1).

Lastly, a final neurological adaptation that occurs when performing heavy work like resistance workouts is that you will also be teaching your motor units to work better in synchronicity, or at the same time. More motor units firing at the simultaneously makes you stronger as you can switch your muscle fibres on at the same time for the strongest possible muscular contraction. This is of course very helpful when you come to lift very heavy loads, as the greatest percentage of your muscle possible will simultaneously be applied to lifting the weight, rather than having different fibres firing in a disjointed and so uncoordinated fashion that would limit your strength, as in untrained people. Hence why exercise also improves coordination.

MORE NERVES FIRING AT THE SAME TIME = GREATER STRENGTH

This is also important for muscular growth. Due to the size variation in the motor units, your muscles will only switch on the type of muscle fibres required for any given task. This switching on process occurs in order in relation to the respective sizes of the motor neurons. So the smallest motor neurons connected to your weakest endurance, or slow twitch muscle fibres, fire first, followed by the different fast twitch fibres up to the fastest, largest and strongest fibres if you lift a heavy enough weight.

What this all means then, is that for quite a long time when you first start doing a new exercise, all you are really doing is learning how to use the muscle mass your body already carries more effectively. You are in essence unlocking the potential strength that has, until now, always been there, but just lying dormant. This period of neurological adaptation has been scientifically proven to take around six weeks ([1]), and must occur for you to be able to maximise your muscular growth in the future.

What you have done in this six week time period, then, is created the key that can now unlock the door to muscular growth. This is why you don't want to make the mistake of thinking that you should skip to a new set of exercises around about now, as too many people do. Otherwise you will be wasting all of the potential for muscle growth that you have just unlocked, since, thanks to the neurological upgrades, if you will, that you have now created, you will now be able to lift heavier weights for longer due to having taught a greater percentage of your muscles to work at the given exercise/s you have been doing. And as seen with the hill example above, now that you have a greater potential for muscular endurance, now you can lift that heavier weight for longer, and move into working in the hypertrophy or growth range for sets in your exercises.

So this is where doing fewer exercises better comes in.

Instead of skipping to a new set of exercises, after six weeks, you will continue to perform the same exercises. This is because whilst the exercise you have been doing may seem easier week-on-week during this period, (hence why you may want to change to different exercises since you may feel they are no longer working), this is mainly just because you are doing the movement more, so are getting used to what it feels like. Basically, the movement has become easier to perform since you are practicing it and so learning to do it better. So initially it is familiarity with the movement that makes the movement seem easier.

But only after giving the suitable amount of time to any exercise will you have reinforced this sense of increasing ease, from an increased familiarity, by forcing your body to make actual changes to your physiology. These changes are the neurological adaptations discussed above. It is these that mean you have now made concrete strength gains through actually reprogramming and so altering your nervous system in a lasting way. These that allow you to actually use a much greater percentage of your existing muscle mass's existing strength potential.

Only once this initial, actual neurological strength adaptation has taken place will you be able to eke every benefit out of the exercises you are doing. For example, you can now concentrate much more on applying other fundamental principles to your workouts, such as using the right form (discussed in Principle 5), and implementing a progressive overload into your training (discussed under Principle 4). Only now then will you actually be poised to start moving onto making other adaptations such as muscle growth to gain further strength.

By now focusing on mastering your form and adding load to the same movements then, you will continue to make neurological adaptations in the correct manner. You will continue to learn to activate as much of the new muscle you are developing as possible as you go forward in your training and so building new muscle. This will best develop not only your maximal strength through greater neurological recruitment and denser muscle fibres with a greater cross sectional area, but also the ability to increase your muscular endurance. (That resistance training improves endurance performance is proven by studies like that by Paavolainen et al. (2)). (If you are interested in why this works, see also Appendix 1.)

To close this section then, I'll quote Reg Park, a man who knew the value of training fewer exercises better like most of those from his day and before, (and also 3 time Mr Universe back in the 1950s and '60s). 'If you want to get bigger, then get stronger!' (If you doubt the validity of their wisdom and what I've presented here, just check out the physiques of people like him and John Grimek).

Safety increases

Perhaps more crucially, the fewer exercises approach will give you the best long term results because it increases exercise safety. This is because you will give your ligaments and tendons time to gain strength alongside your muscles and nervous system, limiting your potential for injury.

Connective tissue strengthening, supported by findings that athletes involved in activities requiring high levels of force exertion have thicker tendons (3), will allow you to apply your strength to your skeleton much more effectively and is another crucial but often overlooked step in developing your strength to its maximum potential. After all, your muscles can only actually exert their new found strength to your skeleton via these connective tissues. Without your connective tissues, your muscles are like a car engine without the chassis—a source that can create power but with no way to transfer that power to the wheels and so actually make the car, or in your case, your body, move.

Basically then, you will only ever be as strong as these connective tissues are, no matter how much you may develop your muscles. This may explain why many body builders (not all), though possessing visually more sizeable muscles than other athletes like powerlifters or gymnasts, often cannot lift anything like as much weight as these athletes, since many don't train with heavy weights but instead just pump their muscles with lighter weights and high reps.

How to still develop your whole body with fewer movements

But how, you may ask, do you develop your whole body with a limited number of exercises? After all, I am telling you to do fewer exercises.

Well, simple. Compound exercises are those in which you move more than one joint to perform a movement. An example is a squat, where your ankles, knees, and hips are moving so that all of your lower body muscles are working to perform the movement.

By contrast, isolation exercises involve moving just one joint to target an individual muscle with the bulk of the load, as in a bicep curl where only your elbow moves. Consequently, far fewer muscles are activated by isolation exercises.

So, to do fewer exercises, all you need to do is perform a low number of compound movements. This way you will still easily be doing an exercise program that works nearly all of your muscles with a minimum number of exercises over the course of a week. This will be shown clearly in the next book in this series dealing with workout programming.

Summary

- Building muscle depends upon first making neurological adaptations that increase your strength
- Only once neurological adaptations have occurred will muscle growth really be promoted so that strength gains continue
- Neurological adaptations that make you stronger through actually altering your body, rather than you just getting more used to or familiar with a movement, take around six weeks to occur
- So you need to perform the same exercises consistently for at least six weeks just to learn to use your existing muscle mass before your body will really start to be able to grow muscle
- As a result, concentrate on doing a limited number of exercises long term
- This will simplify your training so that you can concentrate on more important factors that will give you the results you want whilst still performing the same exercises, like progressive overload
- Since your connective tissues take longer to adapt and grow stronger than your muscles, and these are a vital component in gaining maximal strength, doing fewer of the same exercises but for a prolonged period of time—rather than constantly changing your exercise programs—will also make your training as safe and so effective as possible

Principle 3
Consistent Frequency

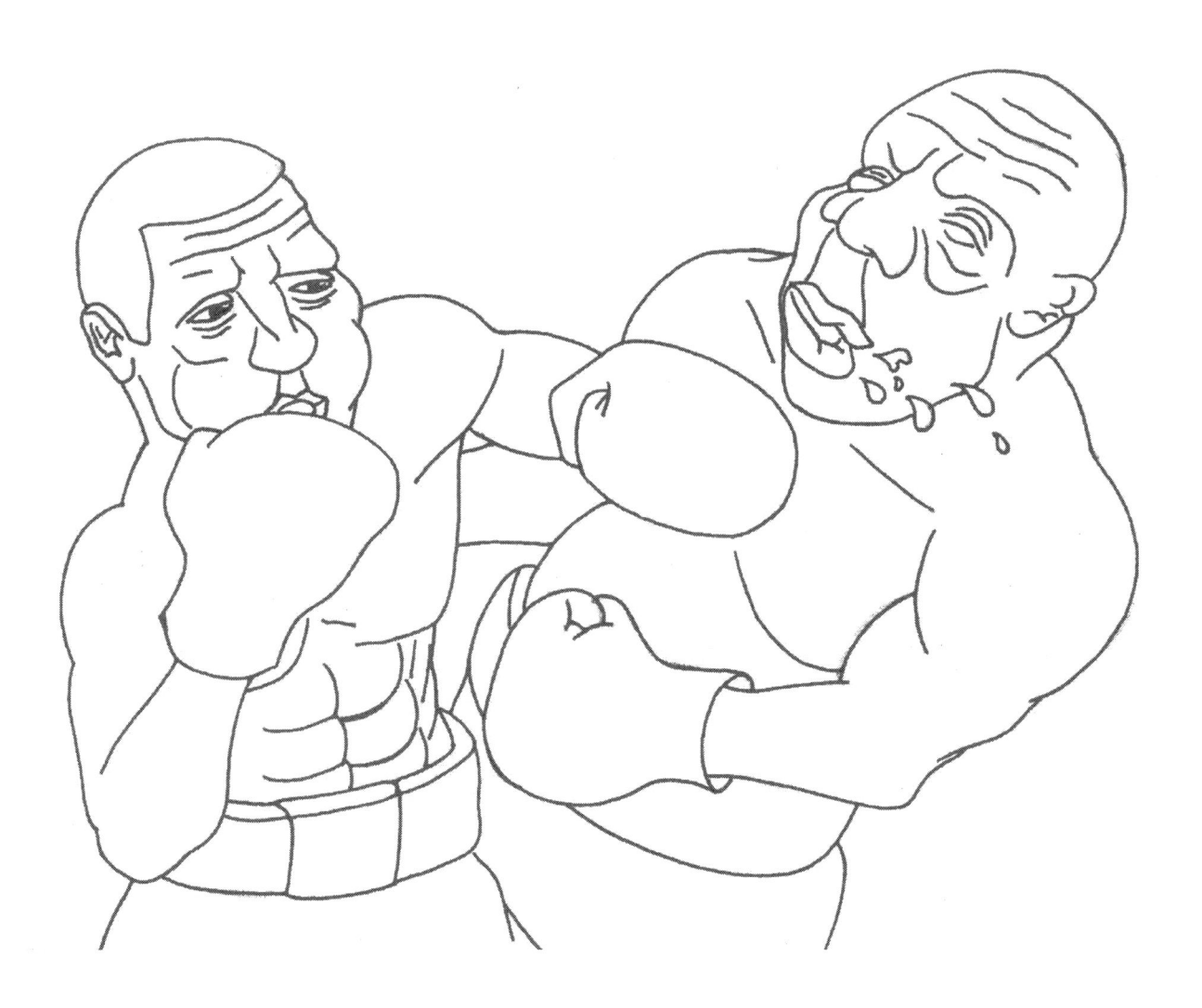

"Success isn't always about greatness. It's about consistency. Consistent hard work leads to success. Greatness will come." Dwayne Johnson

When I mentioned that there is an overabundance of superhumanly strong people on YouTube today, and this can be potentially injurious to peoples exercise goals, what I meant relates specifically to this principle.

All too often, people can look at these people and want to achieve their kinds of levels of strength too soon. So they will jump in with all guns blazing, exercising hard every single day in an effort to make their exercise programs give them results as soon as possible.

Or, on the other side of the equation, people can be disheartened by seeing this kind of phenomenal strength, perhaps thinking they will never be able to achieve such things, so why even bother trying?

But both of these conclusions are a mistake, since exercise needn't be a miserable, full time hobby—providing you approach it correctly, with a consistent frequency, and in a structured way.

Exercising to get the best results is not just about pushing hard every day. Rest is just as important to any exercise program as the exercises themselves, so that you have to balance the exercise that you do with adequate rest. This will allow you to train in a healthy way.

At the same time though, you need to exercise frequently enough to actually get results. After all, you want your exercise to be effective.

Confusing? Contradictory? Well, most likely yes, but what this really means is that by no means do you need to, or, indeed, should you exercise every single day.

How often should you exercise then?

Well, to better explain this, realise that there is a vast gulf between exercise like resistance workouts, and just everyday movement that can still be considered exercise, like walking. This is because of the intensity of the different activities. The harder an exercise type is, the more cautious you need to be with not overdoing it.

So, in the case of walking and just moving in general, doing it every day is a good thing, and highly recommendable. But in the case of harder exercises that are more challenging to your body in terms of recovery time, like resistance workouts, you will need to box smarter to get results, and here's why.

First, understand that the stimulus for your body to improve caused by resistance workouts, or any high intensity workouts, is actually damage caused to your body by the exercises that you do. This damage includes things like micro tears in your muscles. These can only be repaired by new protein synthesis, laying down new proteins, so that your muscles will become denser and stronger. But this can only happen with sufficient rest.

To understand this better, I will need to briefly touch on how muscle cells work to burn energy, to show when improvements from exercise can occur. This will also help to show why too much high intensity exercise can also be damaging if done with an incorrect approach.

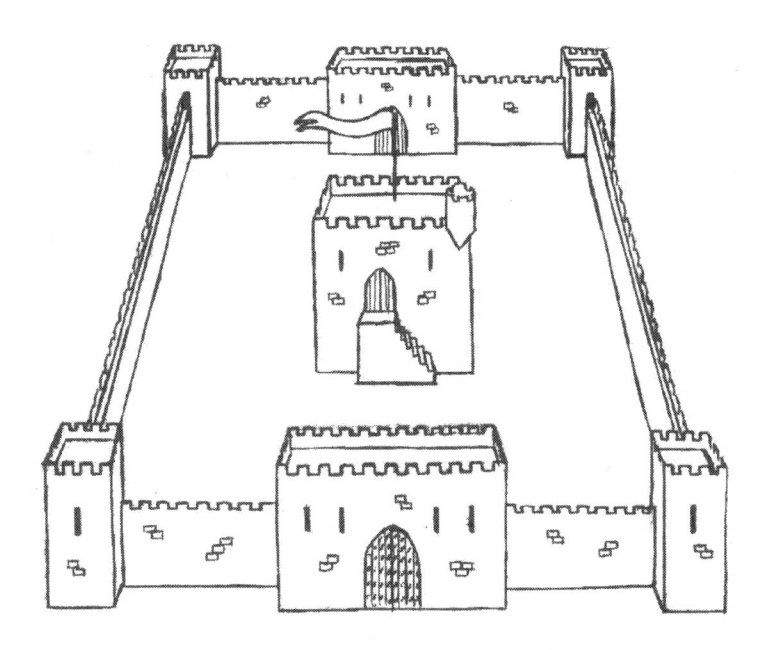

First then, as a really simplified version of muscle cell structure, visualise a muscle cell as being like an old, fortified medieval town in terms of its structure. The fortified wall surrounding the town is the cell membrane, with the gates being the only access points to the cell. The Lord's castle, sitting separately within the town, is the mitochondria of the cell. (Mitochondria are often referred to as the 'powerhouse' of a cell since this is where much of the energy, a molecule called ATP, produced by muscle cells is made.) Finally, all around the Lord's castle but within the fortified walls of the town (the cell), is fluid called cytoplasm (strictly sarcoplasm in a muscle cell).

- Fortified wall = cell membrane
- Town gates = access points to cell
- Lord's castle = mitochondria
- Area around Lord's castle but within fortified walls = cytoplasm/sarcoplasm

Whilst the mitochondria is called the powerhouse of the cell, some energy is also made in the sarcoplasm. But in the sarcoplasm, the cell makes the energy *without* oxygen (anaerobically). In the Lord's castle, this energy, or ATP (Adenosine Tri-Phosphate), is produced *with* oxygen (aerobically).

- Mitochondria (Lord's Castle) = ATP made with oxygen (aerobically)
- Cytoplasm = ATP made without oxygen (anaerobically)

As you can also see from the diagram, to reach the Lord's castle, anything entering the town/cell by the gates first has to pass through the sarcoplasm in order to reach the Lord's castle.

Here's where an important difference between low or moderate, and high intensity activity can occur.

When ATP is made in the Lord's castle (mitochondria), it occurs at a fixed pace. So this form of fuel production can only keep up with low or moderate intensity activity which does not require massive amounts of ATP to be produced in a hurry. This is true of such low intensity activity since you only use your smaller, slow twitch muscle fibres to perform low intensity activities, like steady jogging.

Hard, intense work like resistance workouts, by comparison, need a more rapid source of ATP since this type of workout requires a much greater amount of energy at a much faster pace. This is because your larger, fast twitch muscle fibres are also being worked, and these can only contract for very short periods of time (10-15 seconds in the case of the largest muscle fibres). So they need ATP to be made very rapidly.

The fuel that drives all of this

Understand also that glucose that fuels ATP production can be found both in your blood, so enters the cell via the town gates, but is also stored in your muscle cells and liver already as glycogen.

To best understand how your muscle cells use this glucose then, think of each of your muscle cells as having an energy, or glucose gauge, with 10 being full on the gauge. So your muscle cells can be compared to an energy tank or steam boiler with a full supply of steam ready to power your muscles to move.

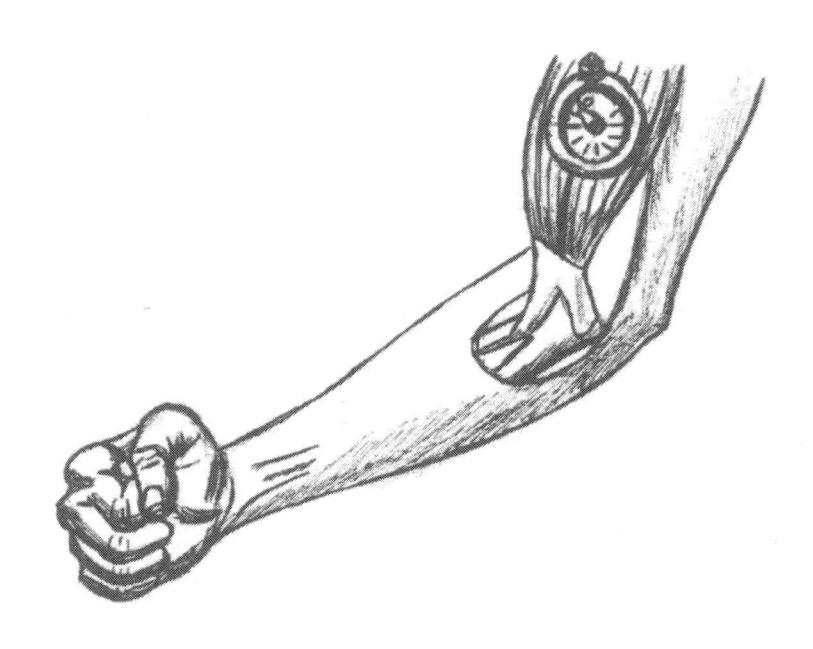

Full gauge, pre workout

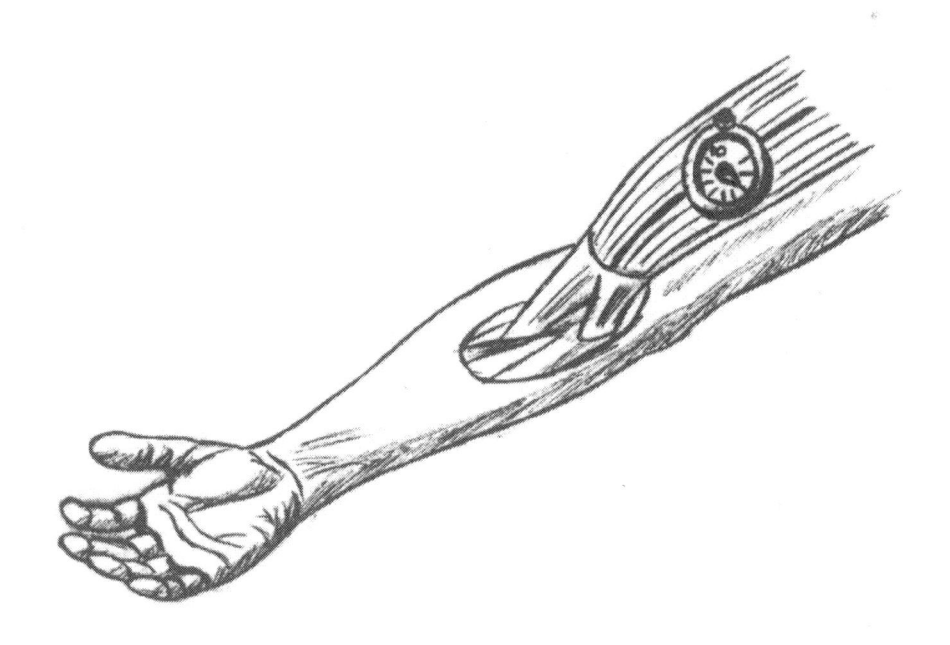

Drained gauge, post workout

Intense exercise drains glucose/energy from your muscle cells much more than low intensity activity. So when you do a hard resistance workout, by the end of the workout the gauge will now show that the energy supply in your muscles has dropped, perhaps to 3, for example.

Here's the important part though. Strength gains and muscle growth can only be developed within your muscles *after* the energy or glucose levels within your muscle cells have again been replenished to the original 10 level on that gauge. Only then are the conditions correct for adaptations like strength increases and growth to occur. So only then is the cell actually able to improve upon its previous level through things like protein synthesis, neurological adaptations, or adaptations for utilising energy more efficiently in the future.

Once adaptations have occurred however, by the standards of the old gauge, your muscle may now be capable of a 13, say, so that your muscle has grown stronger and more able to do a greater level of work in future. According to the gauge analogy then, you are upgrading your muscle's gauge with each workout.

Key to all of this then, as you can hopefully see, is that these improvements or adaptations require time. Your muscle cells must be given time to recoup their energy stores to that 10 level. Additionally though, more time still is required beyond this point for your muscle to improve above that previous level. Time in which the muscle will then be improving in some way so that you are upgrading the gauge.

Here's the whole point of this example though. If you exercise too soon, before your muscles have recovered to this 10 level on the gauge, say to just a 7 on the gauge, you will again drain the muscle cell's levels when you workout again. But after this next workout, you will have dipped even deeper into the muscle's energy tank, since you didn't recover back to at least the 10 level, let alone a higher level, before working out again. So the same level of work as before will now drop the gauge to an even lower level, perhaps a 2, for example. This means extra time still will be required just to return your muscle to its former 10 level, and even more time for any improvement to be made beyond this point.

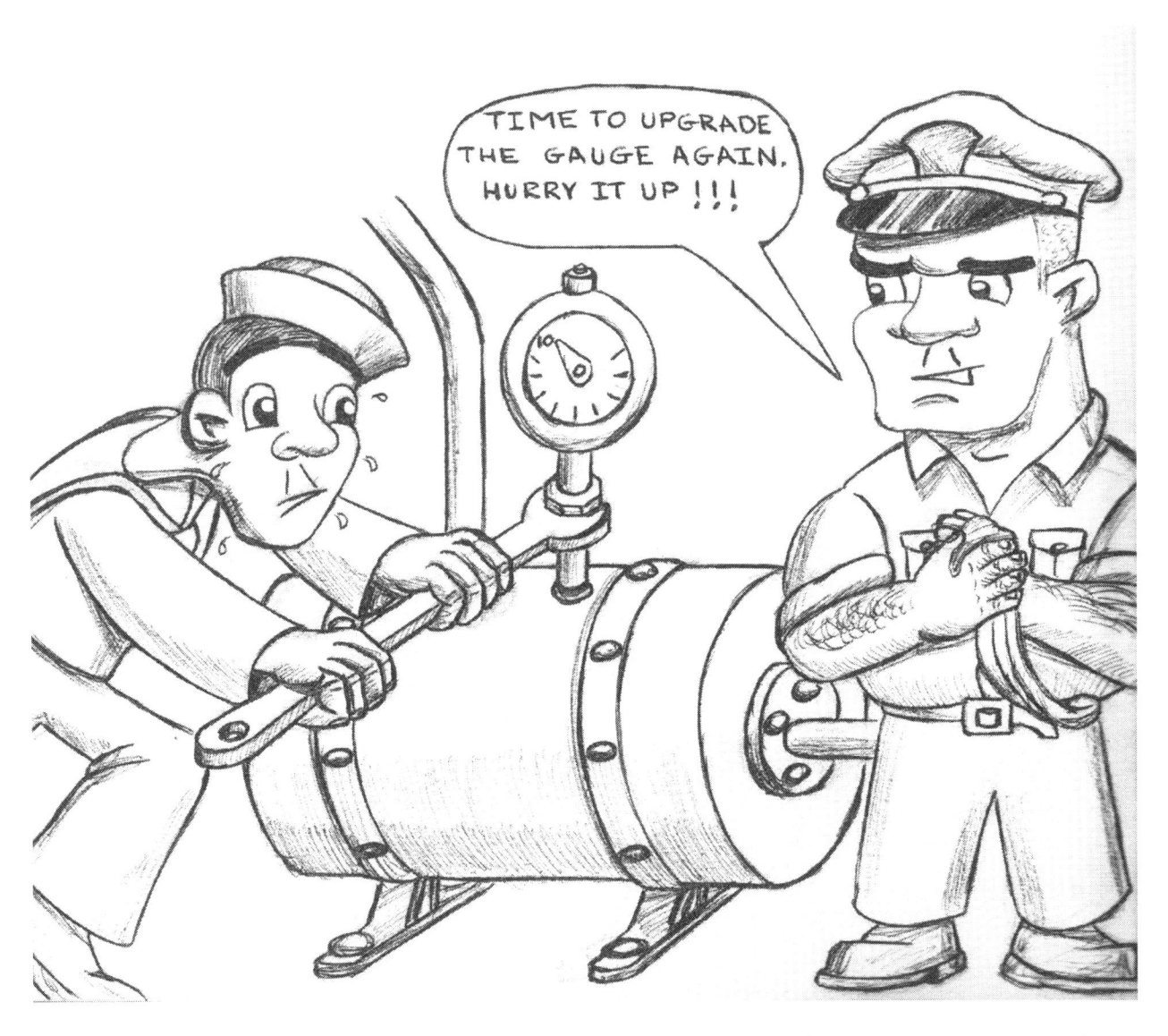

You can see then that this is a sliding scale, with working out too soon only eating deeper and deeper into your ability to recover. Crucially, staying below a 10 level will also prevent you from developing your muscles in any way, since growth and adaptations can only occur once you are back to that 10 level, so that your body can then build upon your previous healthy level. So don't exercise too soon, or you will just rob yourself of any benefits you may be seeking from your workouts.

Worse still, dropping too low will keep you in a constant state of recovery as your body will always be fighting to return your muscle cells to this 10 level. This will place an extra load on your body's systems, so that things like your heart rate will stay excessively high, and long term make you more susceptible to illness. This is a state called overtraining, and the deeper into this state you get, the longer you will need to rest completely to reach that healthy 10 level again. A level that can then take months to return to depending upon how deeply into your energy reserves and recovery ability you have dipped.

So, to put it simply, it is not whilst you are exercising that these adaptations that make you stronger occur, but whilst you rest. So for your body to grow stronger, you have to leave time between your exercise sessions for the repair process to occur. This way, on an ongoing basis, you can keep improving from workout to workout.

Don't push too hard, too soon then, as this will actually just slow your progress through leaving you too sore and stiff, and unrecovered enough to improve from workout to workout.

Consistent Frequency

This is where 'consistent frequency' comes in then, to allow you to benefit most from the exercises you do. But this will inevitably take a little bit of fine tuning at first.

As noted, as well as giving you the best results from your exercise, rest is also essential for your overall, general health, since exercising, just like anything, is actually a bad thing if you do too much of it.

So, you will need to establish just how much rest you, individually, need between each workout.

How to establish the frequency with which you exercise and to which you will consistently stick then?

Well, as you may have guessed, this comes down to intensity, and a process of trial and error regarding this, albeit an informed trial and error. But this will quickly be fine-tuned when you start exercising, since you will learn how to listen to your body with experience (see Principle 7).

Where intensity is concerned, if you always train to failure on your exercises, you are essentially draining that gauge very deeply every time you exercise. Consequently, you will need much more rest between your workouts to ensure that you are fully recovered before exercising again, and to ensure that you are allowing your body to adapt to your training sessions.

As a result, if you train to failure all the time, you will very likely need at least a week between workouts, so that you can only exercise in a resistance workout sense once a week.

Of course, this is not likely to lead to very fast results, however, and let's face it, this is what many people look for. So such an approach will likely prove very unsatisfactory to most.

To get faster results then, particularly in terms of developing high levels of strength, simply never train to failure. This way, you will be able to do many more workouts a week, so that your results will come quicker. (This will be explained in much more detail in *Exercise Programming*, the second volume in this series).

You can also switch between what areas of your body you work through the week, such as upper body one day, lower body the next, to avoid overworking any sets of muscles and so requiring more rest time as a result.

For now though, never training to failure is best achieved by picking a hard enough exercise where you can keep the reps low. By low reps, I mean you should work within the rep ranges per set that are relevant for your current goals. But keep the reps low, away from failure, by always finishing your sets 1 or two reps away from failure. To do this, learn to recognise when your form is deteriorating in any way at all in a given exercise, and stop the set as soon as any loss in form occurs. (For other considerations regarding the point of failure on your exercises, see also Principle 5).

Also, keep the number of sets low. More sets means more of a drain on that gauge and so a greater requirement for recovery time. Again though, this varies depending upon what you are seeking from your training, so that more sets, which means more volume, will lead to greater muscular growth. This can be seen when an easier exercise or load allows more reps to be done towards this end. (See Principle 10 and the *Exercise Programming* book for much more detail,)

In terms of spacing your workouts, the simplest formula to determine how often you exercise and how often you rest, provided you never train to failure, is just to leave at least a day's rest between your workout days. The easiest pattern for this is just to work out three days a week, with four days of rest. This is a sure fire way to be certain that you are getting enough rest since you are getting a day's rest more than you are exercise within each week. Or simplify this still further with two days a week, especially when starting out.

Just as importantly though, a two or three times a week pattern will provide your body with plenty of practice at the exercises you do. This will stimulate your body with an adequate volume of training to induce the adaptations necessary for you to get results from your workouts.

As stated, I will discuss this more in a later book since exercise programming can be made more complex if you work your upper and lower body on separate days, or if you want to do a volume of different exercises that require you to do different exercises on different days of the week to get them all done somewhere in you weekly training. But in the interests of simplicity for now, and especially for beginners or when you have hit a plateau in any particular moves, it is very effective just to limit the exercises you do and to repeat all of these in a single, total body workout done three times a week for the best results, as below.

Just remember, NEVER TRAIN TO FAILURE if using this pattern of workouts or your recovery will assuredly lag.

Exercise 3 x a week example pattern

Mon	Tues	Wed	Thur	Fri	Sat	Sun
Exercise	Rest	Exercise	Rest	Exercise	Rest	Rest

Of course, you can move the days you exercise around the week to best suit you, so long as you always leave a day between workouts, say if you want to exercise on a Tuesday, Thursday and Saturday instead.

Also, here are a few general guidelines that will help you to best set the intensity at which you work, which will have an influence upon your frequency:

- Ideally, you want to feel energized after your workouts. If you feel exhausted after doing a workout rather than better, you are probably working too hard or doing too many exercises within that workout
- You don't really want to be working out for much longer than an hour at a time or ideally 40 minutes or less, since you will likely be tempted to work at a lower intensity level than that which will get you the best results. This is also an easy way to know that you are likely using too many exercises, or just too much volume again
- The longer you take to recover between workouts, the less times a week you can train. But it will be your ability to consistently work out a set number of times a week that will give you the best results. So long term, it is much better to use a greater frequency of shorter, but better quality workouts in terms of intensity each week, than to do fewer, longer, and more draining workouts. If you find that one very good quality workout a week is all you can recover from however, then this is the best training schedule for you. Remember, you have to work to the relevant level for your capabilities

Lastly, realise that any benefits gained from exercise very quickly fade if you stop exercising for any period of time, even within just a few days or a week, unless you have built high levels of muscle and so have a low body fat percentage. But even then your strength will very quickly suffer.

So, *consistency, throughout your life*, is key. *You* alone are responsible for your *own* health and the health of *your* body. So make it a habit to exercise, and it will be far less painful in the long run. In fact, you will likely come to enjoy the process. This is because you should experience far less muscle soreness from doing the same exercises at the correct intensity than by doing all different exercises all of the time, or just working too hard at any given exercise.

Plus you will still have plenty of energy to keep moving in some way every day, which is of course vital to overall health as well.

Summary

- Like anything in life, too much of anything can be a bad thing. So be sure to incorporate adequate rest into your workout programs. We should all be working out to feel better and build ourselves into a

stronger version of ourselves, not to exhaust ourselves. We work out for health, not to break ourselves down to the point of illness, and this very definitely means resting adequately for the results to come
- Exercising 3 x a week will give you a volume of training that will promote the level of practice required to cause adaptations to take place in your body (read adaptations = results)
- A 3 x a week pattern will also allow you to rest for at least a day between each of your workouts, so that balancing rest with exercise is simplified
- But remember, training to failure will increase the amount of time you need to rest between workouts, and so slow your long term results, since you will be able to work out less often a week if you want results and to stay healthy
- The most important thing where workout frequency is concerned is your unique recovery ability, however
- So never be scared to allow yourself extra rest days if you feel too tired to workout, as short term, this will benefit you much more by preventing you from falling into overtraining. After all, overtraining will hinder your long term training, and so cause your results to suffer much more than just shuffling the odd workout around here and there in the short term

Principle 4
Progressive Overload

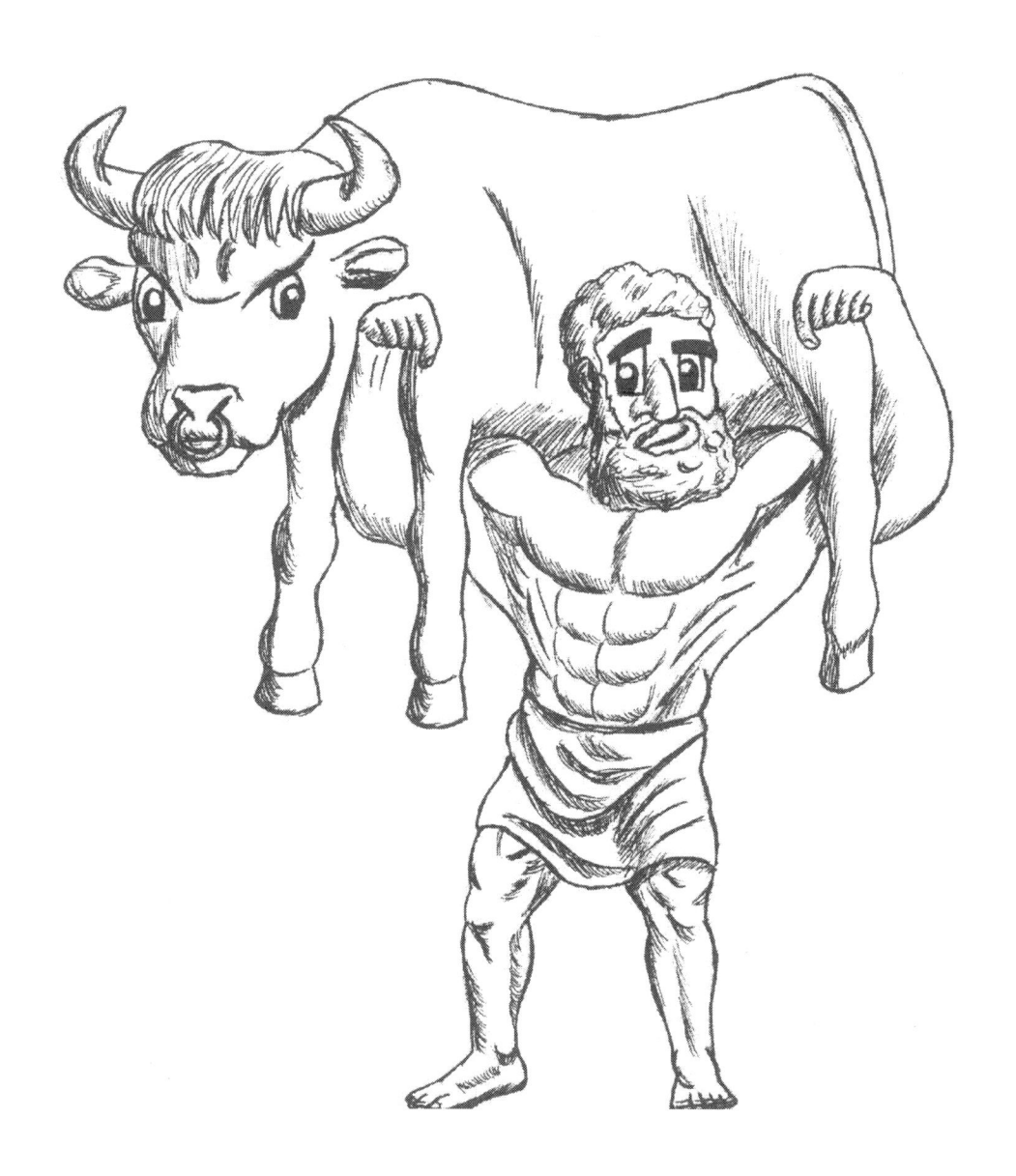

"I am a slow walker. But I never walk back." Abraham Lincoln

This principle relates to a very simple concept that will guarantee that you keep making progress and so advance in your training. But as simple as it is, this is all too often overlooked, so that people stall in their progress and can't understand why they're not growing in size or strength anymore.

So, what is progressive overload?

Progressive means to move forwards or progress in small steps or small degrees.

Overload just means a load that is greater than that which you or something is able to carry. Where this principle is concerned though, it more directly means to use a load that is greater than you *usually* carry. In other words, you lift a weight heavier than that which you are used to handling on a day-to-day basis, or from time-to-time in your workouts. This can be implemented in a number of ways that will be discussed below.

So progressive overload literally means to increase the loads that you work with gradually over time, so in small increments or small steps. In turn, these small steps will then lead to big steps in improvement, like being able to perform a much harder strength position in the long run than you can at present, or a much harder strength movement. With bodyweight exercises then, you move through the progressions, so may move from kneeling push-ups to full-push-ups; full push-ups to archer-push-ups and so on and so forth.

This causes the body to consistently work at a level above that which it is accustomed to, which forces the body to consistently adapt to these higher levels of work. Resultantly, you will, over time, grow stronger, bigger muscles, as your body adapts to the new challenges being placed upon it.

Very important to note here though is that the *gradual* nature of this principle is absolutely fundamental. As mentioned in Principle 2, neurological adaptations can take 6 weeks or longer to occur, so you can only really keep pushing to higher levels of work to a significant extent every six weeks or even longer.

Whilst you want to be progressing over time then, don't just fall into the trap of thinking you can increase your workload substantially every week for the fastest possible results. This will just tire you out prematurely and potentially lead to injury or overtraining, as discussed under Principle 3.

Progressive overload has to be implemented with a plan, such as periodisation (explained in Principle 8). When linked with doing fewer exercises better and periodisation though, progressive overload will be your best path towards success.

To build progressive overload into your workout programs, you can vary any of the following.

1. Load: This is the easiest method, since you simply lift more weight, or, as with bodyweight exercises, use a harder progression of a bodyweight exercise. This way, a higher percentage of your bodyweight is focused upon the targeted muscle group or groups that you are working
2. Intensity: This really refers to the level of effort that you put into an exercise. Of course, if you use a heavier load, so a higher percentage of your 1 rep max load, you should put more effort into your exercises automatically. But this isn't necessarily the case if you lack focus and so still do an exercise incorrectly. Intensity then really comes down to correct effort through using good form and mental focus to really contract your muscles with your maximum effort. The higher the effort, the more benefit you will get in terms of strength gains. A good example of this is forcing your muscles to work with more effort on a momentary basis and so a greater intensity through slowing your reps down. This would be the case if you did the lowering portion of a push-up for 4 seconds, then hold the bottom position for a second, before rising up explosively and doing all of your repetitions like this instead of just pumping out fast push-ups. (Various approaches are covered in more detail in Principle 9)
3. Volume: This relates to accumulated load. In other words, any way that you do a greater total amount of work within a workout, so by increasing:

    - Reps: Simply performing more reps of an exercise over time will make you stronger since you will lift a greater cumulative load. This will make your cumulative intensity greater through using a greater overall effort. This is also an easy way to visibly see that you are growing stronger. (See Principle 10 for rep ranges to target different areas of development, whether strength, growth or muscular endurance)

- Sets: When you are able to do your target reps in a single set of any exercise, start to add sets so that you simply multiply how many times you perform this number of reps, thus increasing the total load you lift during your workout through again increasing the volume of work

4. Rest Periods: You can also reduce the rest periods between sets, to make the exercise more intense. This intensity increase will mainly apply to metabolic stress ($_4$), (a variable in muscular growth), so that the accumulation of waste products in your muscles will become a limiting factor. If you want to build strength as well as muscular size though, your rest periods should ideally be around 2 minutes long or shorter. So don't rest any longer than this, and ideally for 3-5 minutes if focusing upon strength development. (Longer rest intervals limit the metabolic stress, allowing you to work harder and so to target strength more)

Any of these variables can be used to implement a progressive overload into your workouts. Whether you implement these steps over long periods or from workout-to-workout, or week-to-week is up to you, as we all develop differently. Just be sure to work to your own schedule, remembering that *gradual progress* trumps racing ahead too soon, so always be careful about pushing to failure by trying to implement any of these steps too soon. Remember, whilst you may feel you are progressing faster by doing more reps each workout, as an example, if you are also tiring yourself too much, long term you are actually slowing your progress down. (See Principle 3).

If adding reps feels like you will be pushing close to failure, add an extra set of a few reps or however many are one short of that failure point. Or better still, stick with the same reps/sets, and just add a little more intensity by slowing the exercise down, but again being careful to stop one rep short of failure, even if this means doing fewer reps initially.

- For max strength, add intensity, like slowing down your reps, ideally within the 1-5 rep range
- For more size, add reps within the 8-15 rep range

Also, make sure that you are using this principle regularly, in any of the above ways, applied to the same exercises for the sake of simplicity, and you cannot fail to improve your physique in terms of muscular development and strength increases. These things, and not the exercises you do, are the only aspects of your workout program that you need to vary in order to keep making progress whilst also preventing the headache of overcomplicating things. *Simple is best.*

Summary

- Progressive overload must be included into your training in some regard for your training to keep giving you cumulative results long term. So over time, you must incorporate adjustments to any of the following:
    - Load
    - Intensity or effort
    - Volume—reps and sets
    - Alteration of rest periods

Principle 5
Correct Form
Focus upon this before anything else

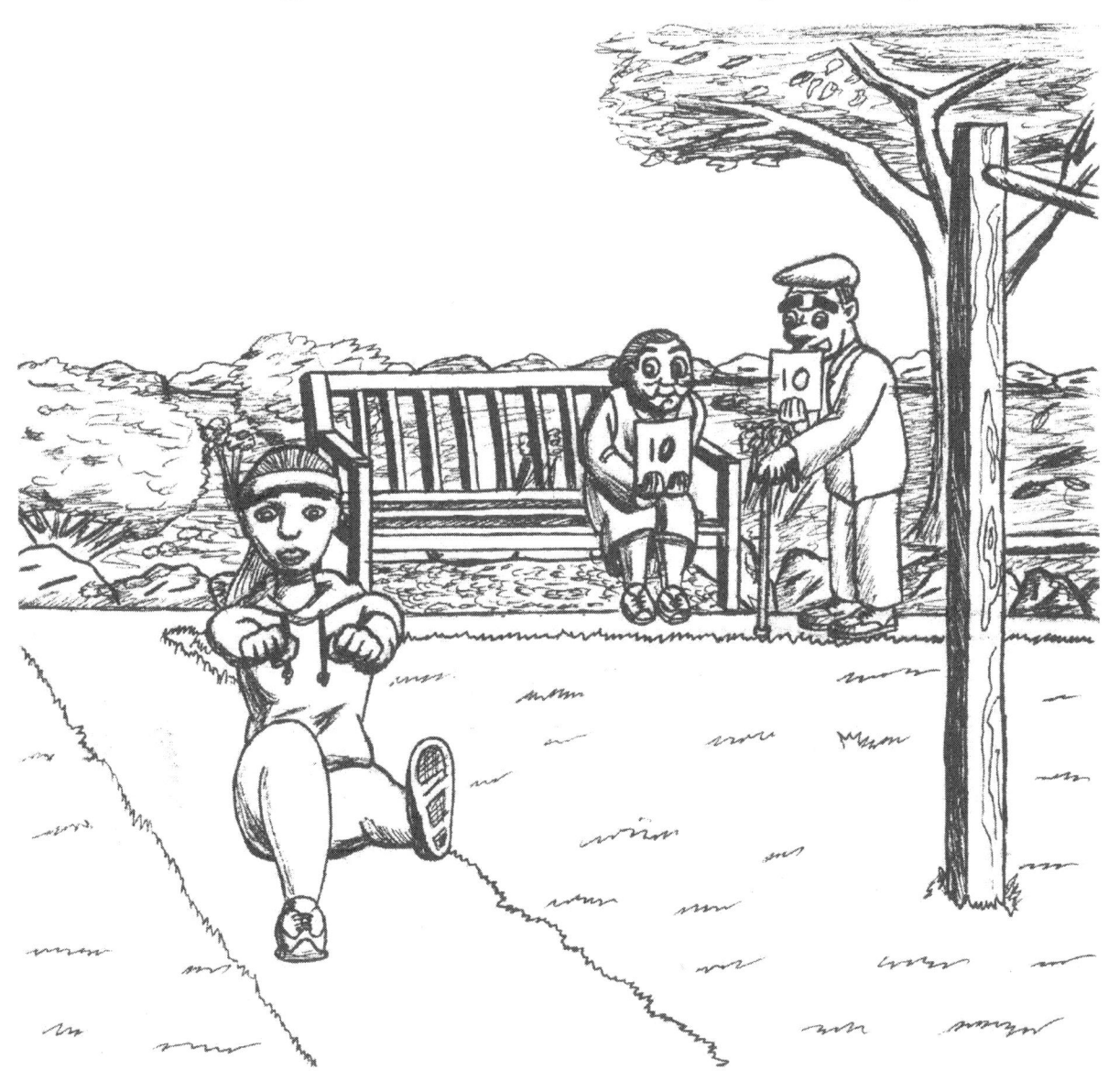

"Practice does not make perfect. Perfect practice makes perfect." Vince Lombardi Jr.

Correct form is fundamental when you exercise for the following reasons:

- It ensures your joints are aligned and loaded correctly. This makes an exercise as safe as possible, limiting the potential for injury
- Maximum activation of the muscles involved in the movement. This means that you will get the best results in all regards
- Correct stimulation and so development of your nervous system. This means that good habits when moving will be programmed into your body both during exercise, but also in all daily activities, so that you can apply your developing strength in an intuitively correct manner

This principle may seem very obvious, but is far too often ignored or abused. This is probably because everyone equates volume with results, since doing something more is perhaps the easiest way to perceive that you are making improvements.

But again, going back to the simplicity equals mastery theme, you should absolutely focus on the basics at all times, and maintaining good form throughout all of your repetitions is perhaps the most fundamentally basic rule you should adhere to at all times. After all, doing anything lots of times inevitably leads to a drop in focus, and so a drop in quality and effort. And where exercise is concerned, quality and effort absolutely trumps quantity.

So, focus on doing each repetition correctly throughout the length of your workouts. The moment your form starts to deteriorate, stop the exercise, even if this means doing far fewer repetitions than usual. Doing even two or three repetitions absolutely correctly is far better than doing ten repetitions badly. More reps but with bad form will just lead to injury sooner or later, and disappointing results overall.

Understand that a point of failure on any exercise doesn't just mean a point at which you will collapse if you do another rep then. Failure should be counted as being unable to do another rep with absolutely correct form.

Remember, strength development is as much, if not more, about training your nervous system than it is about building bigger muscles. Therefore strength development is skill development. So treat it like any other skill, where the pursuit of excellence is the goal. Doing repetitions with poor form takes away the excellence, and renders the exercise a waste of time.

Work to perfect your exercises just like you do any other skill then. Don't settle for anything less than perfection and your results will reflect this.

Summary

- It is far better to do fewer reps better in terms of form and effort applied to them, than doing lots of reps with bad form
- Treat your exercise like developing any skill, so that you aim to perfect the skill with regular practice
- The second your form breaks down, stop the exercise short there, so that this is your failure point on that exercise, when you think about doing your reps to failure

Principle 6
Mental Focus
Using the mind to improve your results

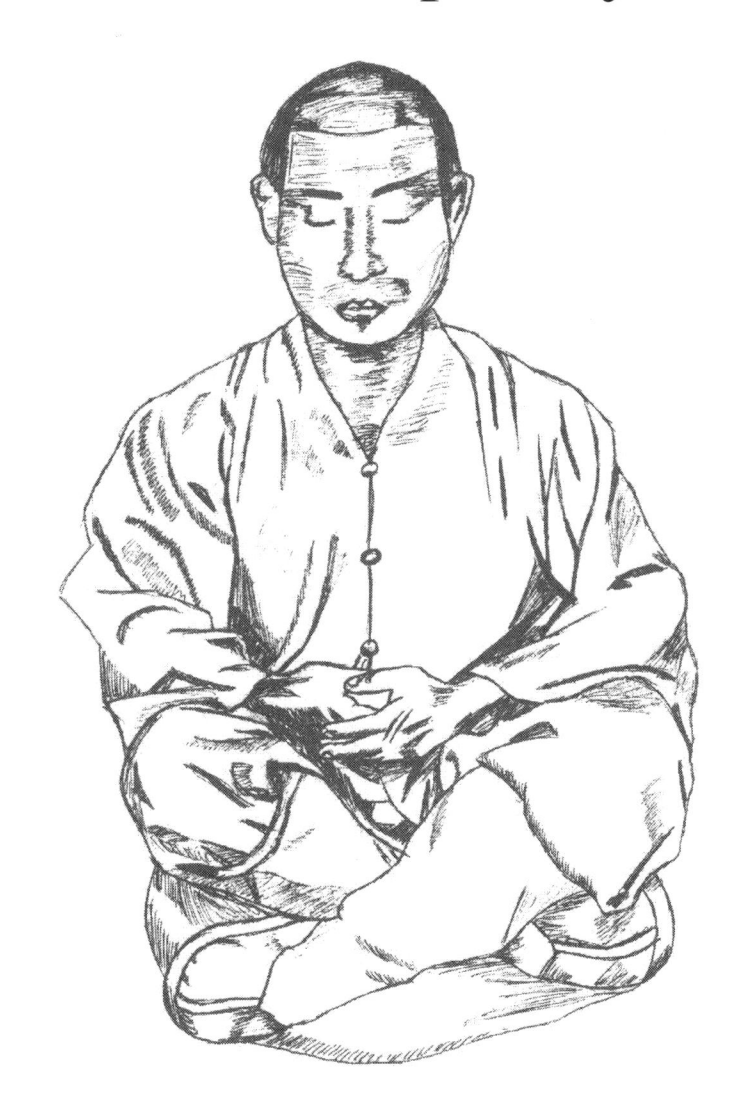

"The mind is the limit. As long as the mind can envision the fact that you can do something, you can do it, as long as you believe 100 per cent."

Arnold Schwarzenegger

If you have already been a regular exerciser for any length of time, you may have heard of the idea of what is often called a mind-to-muscle connection when you work out. This is an idea bodybuilders have used for a long time, whereby they literally focus their mind upon the muscle or muscles they are working whilst performing a given exercise. Indeed, in some cases, they speak of talking to the muscles they are working, even telling these muscles to grow.

This may seem a little bit strange. Why the hell would you talk to your muscles after all? But this isn't so much a case of *talking* to the muscles contracting to perform an exercise, but more a case of placing your *mental focus* upon the muscles that are working. This means that you are fully focused upon what you are doing, and therefore concentrating upon what you want the outcome of the movement you are performing to be. This will in turn make your exercises much more effective since you can devote far more effort to the movement, and if you have to use the mental cue of actually imagining speaking to your muscles, well, then all well and good, since this will just make you consciously aware of your thoughts.

But why should this work?

In scientific terms, because you have two branches of your nervous system: a conscious, or voluntary, and an unconscious, or involuntary branch. This is because some actions, like keeping your heart beating, must be beyond your control, or else you would constantly be occupied with telling your heart to beat.

Your involuntary nervous system also controls reflex actions like blinking to protect your eye, so that these movements are also reflexive rather than voluntary. On some levels though, even conscious actions, like performing an exercise, can seem like involuntary actions in the regard that you apply minimal amounts of actual conscious thought to conducting these movements.

In a sense then, through a lack of concentration, you can essentially remove your brain from the action, or do a movement mindlessly and so far from to the best that you potentially can.

To demonstrate this, try this quick experiment, applied to clenching your fist. (The idea behind this exercise is inspired by similar awareness exercises I first came across in a book by Peter Ralston called *Zen Body-Being* (5). I absolutely recommend reading this eye-opening book where physical potential is concerned.)

Think to yourself now, how often do you actually try to feel what your hand is doing whilst you clench your fist, rather than just going through the motions? By this, I mean how often do you actually analyse what it really feels like to clench your fist, in terms of what each part of your hand feels like during this movement?

This is quite a diffuse idea to explain so to better understand what I mean, go ahead and clench you fist now.

No doubt you clenched your fist, with very little thought put into the movement, since you know how to clench your fist, right?

So what you just did when you clenched your fist is akin to the unconscious manner in which your body can breathe without you having to think about doing so. In other words, although there was obviously an element of your mind telling your hand to clench, you nonetheless clenched your fist in as unconscious and as automatic a manner as possible since you didn't really have to think about clenching your fist.

Now, unclench your fist, but this time when you clench your hand again, keep your fist clenched and place all of your mental focus on that fist. Think about what each individual finger feels like, what each part of each finger feels like. Do the same with your thumb. With your palm. With the top of your hand; your knuckles. Really concentrate on what each part of your hand feels like.

What should hopefully result from this is a kind of very heightened sensory awareness of what each part of your hand actually feels like. An awareness that shows you very clearly that you are now absolutely consciously thinking about your hand and how you have clenched your fist. This approach is more akin to the way that you can consciously take control of your breathing, where you actually tell yourself to take each breath so that your breathing has become a voluntary action. And this is exactly what is meant by a mind-to-muscle connection: an actual mental awareness of what your body is doing.

This means the *conscious* aspect of your brain is very much in *conscious* or voluntary control and aware of your movements.

If this is hard for you, keep practicing this same simple exercise until you start to experience a heightened level of mental focus and so connection between your brain—your mind—and your fist. Because this is an example of what you should eventually be doing during all exercises that you perform, and as always, practice makes perfect.

So tell me now, when have you ever felt a connection, like in the above exercise, between your mind and the muscles that you know should be contracting to perform whatever exercises it is that you do? When have you ever felt how tense or relaxed individual muscles are during any exercise to this degree?

The answer for many of you will likely be very rarely.

This is because the human body is, if you like, the ultimate survival machine, as indeed are all living organisms. What I mean by this is that your body is only too happy to put the absolute minimum effort into producing a desired outcome that you ask it to achieve, since evolution has hotwired all of us to use as little energy as possible so that survival is as certain as possible. So if your body can find a way to cheat a movement like an exercise to make it easier to perform, by only minimally contracting the muscles working to produce that desired movement, it will absolutely do so.

For this reason, the kind of mindless training many people do, where they are not focusing wholeheartedly upon each movement they are performing, and just literally have the diffuse mind set of, 'I am going to do a pull-up', say, is far from the optimal approach. This mindless approach akin to just clenching your fist unconsciously because I told you to, as in the first example of the clenching your fist exercise laid out above. In fact, because of such mindless training, many people doing pull-ups don't even know how to engage their back muscles to perform the movement, and instead make this an arm dominant move. Even though pull-ups are very definitely supposed to be performed with your back muscles first and foremost, and your arms are secondary muscles, if you like, that transfer the power of your back to the bar.

This is exactly because of the easiest is best approach that your body likes. If you just try to do exercises on a wholly physical basis, with only general thought directed towards doing the exercise and no conscious thought from you mind applied to the muscles employed in the movement, you are allowing your body to take the easy way out. You are literally cheating yourself out of the majority of the results that you could otherwise gain from each exercise, since your body is operating in close to an unconscious mode. Consequently, your effort level will be far lower than it could potentially be if you start practicing your movements with this mind-to-muscle approach.

So to get the best results from your exercises, you need to be the one consciously controlling each movement. This comes back to many of the other principles, like the need to keep good form, which again is borne from consciously placing your body in the right position. This requires a level of consciousness about what the parts of your body are doing.

It also means that you need to learn what muscles each exercise is working, so that you can learn to contract these muscles maximally, and you need to do this by consciously thinking about the muscles you want to contract.

At first, applying this during your exercises may very well be too challenging since this is something most of us rarely do. But if you just sit and think about the muscle(s) you want to gain control of, telling them to contract through an awareness of where they lie in your body, over time this will become much easier. Especially if you try to consciously practice this at least a few times a day.

All of this, then, will allow you to perform the exercises you do as perfectly as possible. This will give you as much control and muscular activation as possible, so that you get the absolute best results from each exercise. This will prevent you from wasting much of your time. Something you will certainly be doing when you exercise unconsciously, with a minimal amount of effort.

This adds more detail to what I touched upon in the previous principle then, about approaching your exercise as skill practice. Approach each exercise session as practice to acquire a new skill, focusing your mind only on what you are doing and the muscles involved, and in the long run your exercise sessions will become much more productive and rewarding in terms of both the physical results you gain, and the improved mental focus you will attain.

And of course, with practice, this will all come more naturally. In time, this will itself become akin to a reflex action when you call upon your body to employ the strength you develop in your exercise in daily activities, with the outcome that you will become a much more coordinated person.

Summary

- You should never treat your mind and your body as separate entities
- To get the best results from your exercise, realise that the effort and focus of your mind can absolutely increase the level of physical effort that you can apply to each exercise
- So use mental focus to maximize your physical efforts which will in turn maximize your results

Principle 7
Patience
Learn to listen to *your* body

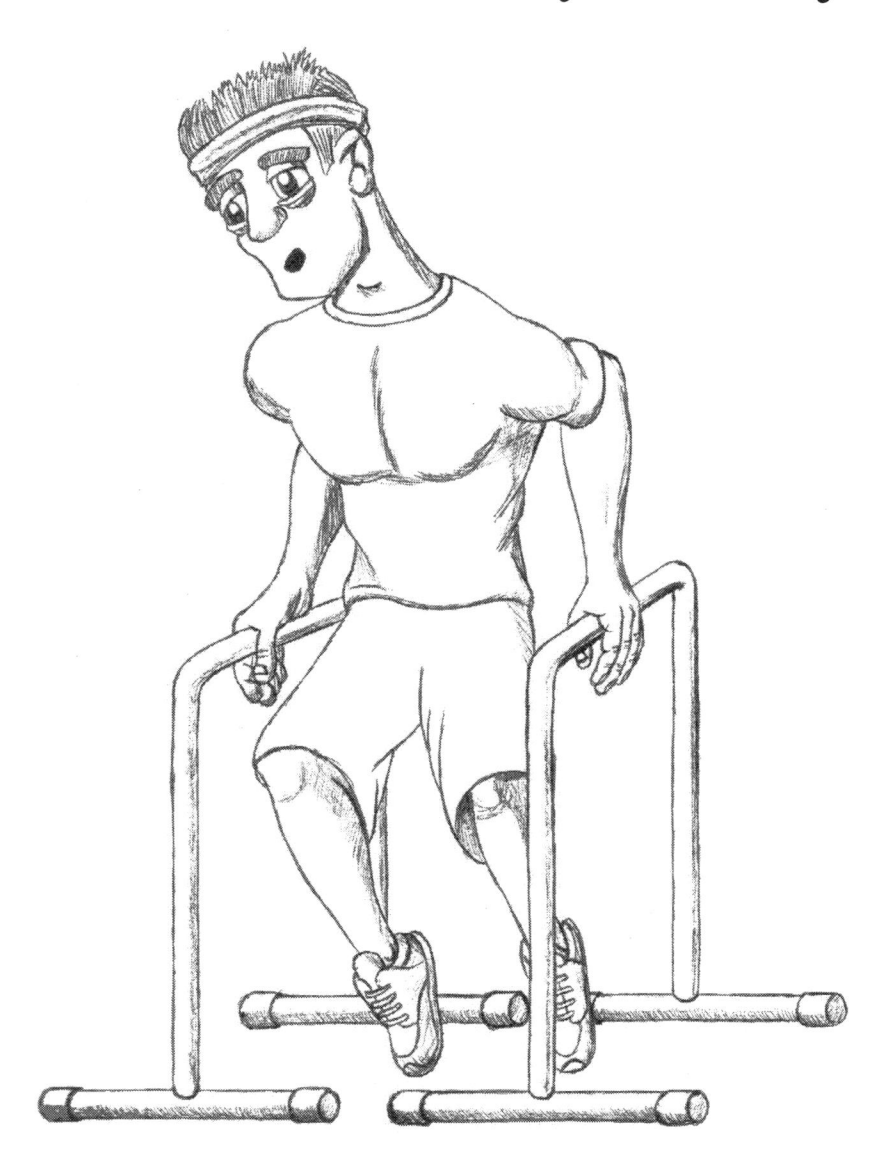

"The greatest wealth is health." Virgil

Whenever we embark on any exercise program, we want to get results. More often than not, we also probably want to get these results fast, hence why the internet is plastered with exercise related advertising that targets achieving results within a set time period—the 'get a six pack in six weeks' kind of ploy. After all, the people espousing these things know this sells.

However, patience is also a key principle in any exercise program, at least any one that is actually going to work. This links back to Principle 1 and SMART, where one of the pointers for goal setting is to be realistic, and also Principle 3: Consistent Frequency.

Don't let yourself fall prey to false promises about unrealistically fast gains being possible. Only time and effort devoted towards a well thought out exercise program, with solid principles at its core will get you the results you want. Hence why the idea discussed in Principle 4 in this book is called *progressive* overload. Remember, progressive means progress made through small steps leading to big improvements for progress to be made. This of course takes time, but will absolutely work.

Patience is important then because it will give you the necessary will power to stick to your program. After all, consistency is where results will be won.

More importantly though, progress, being gradual, will be achieved in a safe manner. Impatience is what leads to using too heavy a load too soon, and this will only lead to injury and delaying your progress since you may have to stop exercising full stop for a time. This is not the way forward. Remember, be honest with yourself and your current level, since small, but consistent gains over time will be the most successful path towards the results you want to achieve in the long run.

A big part of developing this necessary patience is, as such, learning to listen to your own body. By this, I mean that only you live in your own body, so only you can be the real judge of how you actually feel on a day-to-day basis, or know what level of strength you currently possess.

So if, on the day of your workout, you don't necessarily feel as strong as usual for whatever reason, or you know full well that you have a niggling injury, you must take responsibility for managing this. Whether this be by just exercising at a lower level than usual, with fewer reps or sets, as an example, or by skipping a particular exercise that may agitate the niggling injury you suspect exists, or skipping a workout altogether, you must learn to employ the right solution dependent upon your own body at any point in time. Or, you must acknowledge that a particular progression of an exercise is too hard for you at the current time. This will ensure you don't do that exercise with bad form and so run the risk of injuring yourself.

Of course, this doesn't mean that this is an excuse to skip workouts through laziness or just a lack of motivation. Again, these are things you must face yourself and be responsible and accountable for, holding yourself to your course of action.

No, learning to listen to your body is more about maintaining the ability to keep improving long term. After all, if you aren't exercising to stay healthy long term but only to try and look good, you're missing a massive slice of the benefits that come from staying fit. Namely, the ability to lead an elevated quality of life throughout your life, not just for part of it.

Essentially then, this principle is about maintenance through looking after yourself and keeping yourself as healthy as possible, since this is, after all, why you are exercising in the first place—to make yourself healthier. This includes preventing injury and of course illness, which can result if you keep pushing too hard and thus run yourself into the ground through overtraining (as explained in Principle 3).

Don't just passively rely on incorporating rest into your workout programs to ensure that you are training in a healthy manner then. You also have to learn to actively listen to what your own body is telling you so that you learn to recognise when you are fully recovered from a previous workout. Forget about your ego and be honest with what you can actually achieve at any given time. Only this way will you be able to continue to exercise consistently and so effectively.

Summary

- Just adding rest days between your workout days is a good passive way to ensure that you are balancing rest with your exercise to get the best results

- But you also have to learn to actively listen to what your body is telling you on a day-to-day basis
- Use this learned awareness to tell you about things like your energy levels, how tired you may or may not be, and whether you have any niggling injury issues. Use this to adjust your training as necessary during any given workout

Principle 8
Periodisation
Balancing exercise with rest and recovery

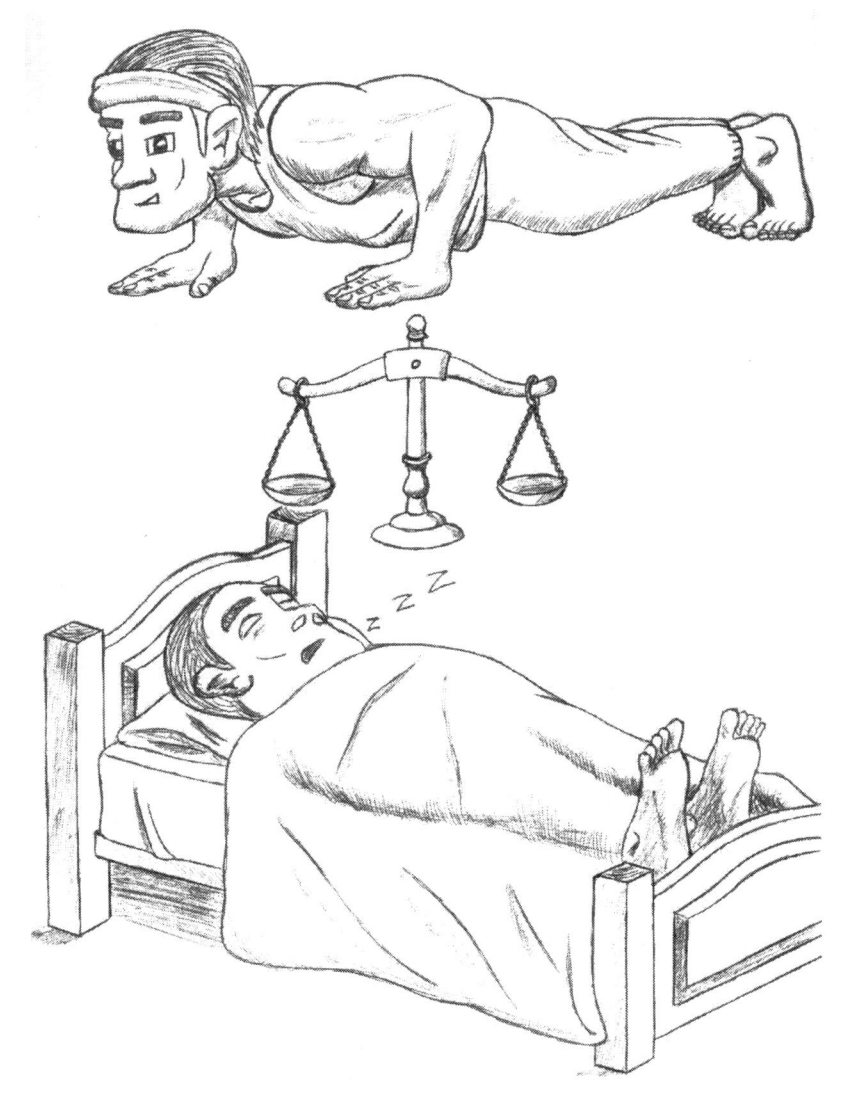

"Fatigue is the common enemy of us all—so slow down, rest up, replenish and refill."

Jeffrey R. Holland

Using periodisation in your training also relates to how you structure the pattern of your workouts over time, much like Principles 3 and 7, which will be key to informing this process. But more specifically, periodisation is how you structure your exercise over the longer term, so over weeks and months rather than just within a single week.

So periodisation will require you to establish a pattern for how many times a week you exercise, and also for how many weeks at a time—the overall work period. This period is how long you exercise for continuously before you require a longer rest or recovery period than just the days you leave between each of your workouts.

Such a rest or recovery period will consist of either a rest week, where at the end of your workout period you will not do any of your workouts for a whole week, or a de-load week.

A de-load week differs from a rest week because it is an active rest. This means you will still do your workouts, but at a much reduced intensity. So you might do:

- half as many sets and reps
- reduce the weight that you use
- do an easier version of a bodyweight exercise
- all aimed at working at a level of intensity around 50 to 60% of your normal workouts

So a de-load week will allow you some rest since you are working at a level of effort or intensity far below that which your body is now more used to working at during your work periods. But this holds the benefit over a complete rest week of reducing the possibility of losing too many of the benefits gained from your exercise period by not exercising at all for a week. So a de-load week is usually the better way to incorporate rest into your exercise cycles.

Again though, employ Principle 7, and listen to your body to decide if you need an absolute rest or just a reduction in workload from period-to-period, remembering that not resting enough will be just as harmful, if not more so, than resting too much. The same applies for the number of days between your workouts if you have pushed too hard. Remember, never be afraid of adding as many days as you feel are necessary for your energy levels to come back to normal before exercising again.

An example of this principle then would be to exercise for six weeks (your overall work period), incorporating a progressive overload so that perhaps from week-to-week, you are pushing to improve in some way, to ensure you are working at a high enough intensity. If to maintain the level of effort you can exert during an exercise you need to stick to working at the same level however—say doing the same number of reps or sets for longer than you have scheduled for in your goals—that is fine too. After all, only if you can maintain good form whilst adding reps or sets should you do so, so use your form as a guide to know when you increase your work load in some way, remembering that quality is better than volume done badly.

Recognise then that the number of weeks you exercise for before ending the cycle and having a rest or de-load week is dependent upon yourself. It will be built around the pattern of weeks that works best for you, in terms of ensuring you are neither too tired to do your usual daily activities like work, and also in terms of making the best steady progress. As you gain experience of what you are capable of, you can also use this to start improving your ability to set yourself realistic goals for each work period.

Consequently, the length of your work periods before taking a rest or de-load week may take a little trial and error to establish at first, but will be worth discovering so that you understand what frequency of training works best for you long term. (Don't think the training volume has to be 3 x a week. That is, remember, just an example. Again, use your own discretion based on what you feel capable of).

Also, as you progress in your training over time, realise it will also be a certainty that you will start to get less results over time. This is just a natural part of any exercise program, particularly a resistance exercise program, since there is only a limited length of time in which you can really keep increasing the workload in a substantial way. After this, your improvements will inevitably become smaller and take longer to achieve.

Basically then, the stronger you get, the harder it will become to still make substantial gains as you will inevitably be reaching your limits and so only be able to increase the load you lift more gradually. (This applies to hypertrophy too. A study by Always et al. (6), for example, showed that in bodybuilders that had been training for more than 5 years, there was no muscular growth in their biceps after 24 weeks of training, demonstrating how hypertrophy also inevitably slows with time.)

A result of this will also likely be that the stronger you get, the longer you may need to rest between your workouts to keep making progress. After all, remembering back to Principle 3, the stronger you get, the greater the fuel tank of your muscles' cells gets (the gauge gets upgraded). This also means you become better at draining this tank however, since you grow stronger, so will be working at increasing intensities and so potentially draining your fuel tank more deeply in each workout. So monitoring your intensity at all times remains a necessary skill that grows in importance the stronger you get.

Don't find this disheartening or a problem though, as you will still be able to make improvements to your body and so get results. It will just mean that your progress will inevitably, but unavoidably slow, and you will have to learn to train smarter. This will require the use of techniques like cycling, which will be explained in a later book (*Bodyweight Exercise: Exercise Programming*).

Summary

- For best results when you train long term, you need to divide your training into periods consisting of a cumulative number of weeks in a row of training
- In between these periods of training, you will likely need to incorporate longer periods of rest than just the rest days that you incorporate between your workout days, depending on the intensity of your workouts and how well you can control this
- These rest weeks can be a total rest where you do no workouts, or more effectively a de-load week at 50-60 % of your usual workload
- Whether you use a rest week or a de-load week will depend upon you as an individual and how you feel at any given point in your training
- The results you can get from your exercise programs will inevitably slow down over time, so that it will become harder to keep improving, but by no means impossible
- Be conscious of the fact that the stronger you get, the longer you may find you need to rest between workouts in order to recover fully

Principle 9
Different Approaches
Eke out every gain from each exercise

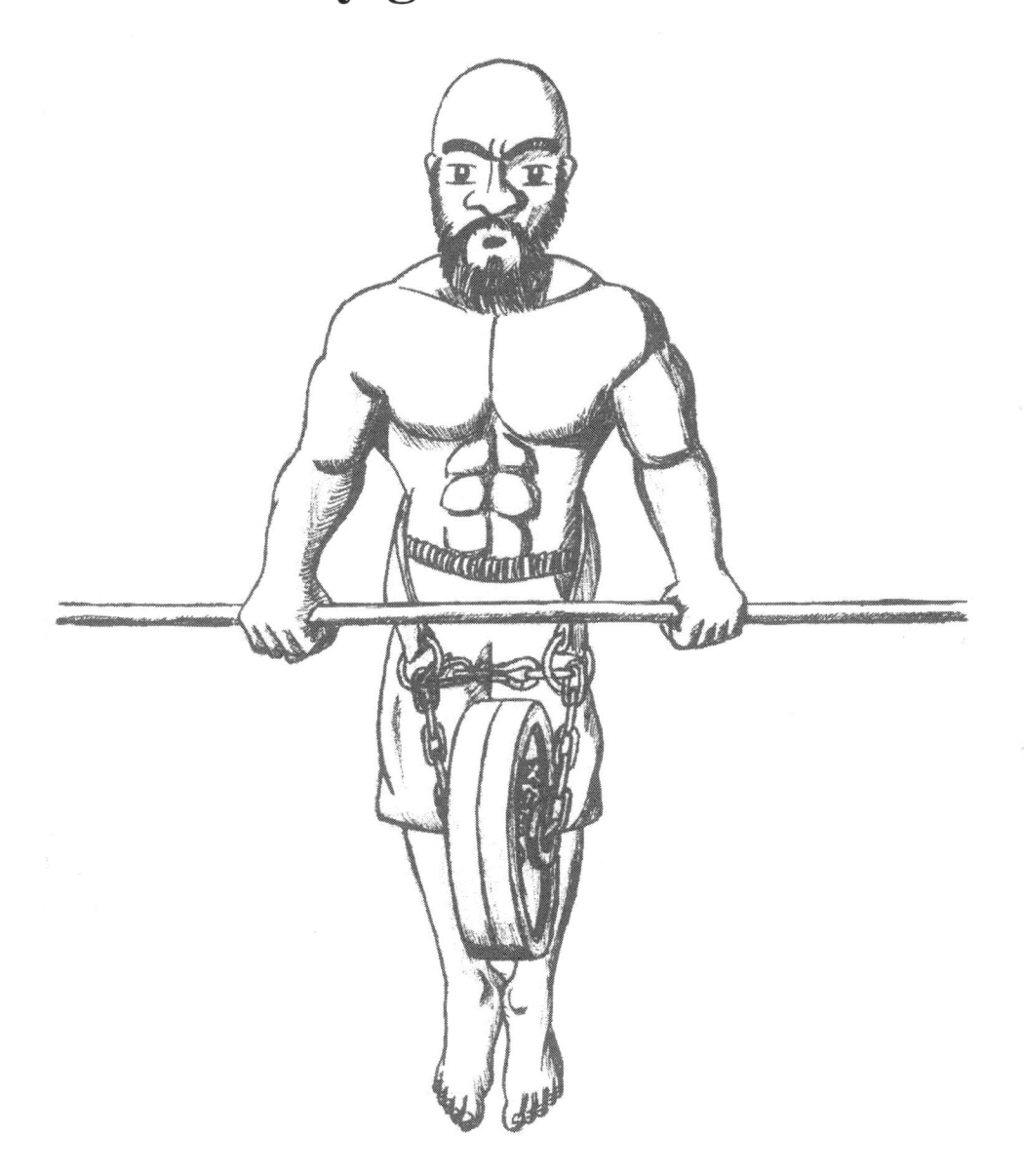

"Impossible is just a word thrown around by small men who find it easier to live in the world they've been given than to explore the power they have to change it." Muhammad Ali

When using any exercise program, even one with fewer exercises done better, you will inevitably find yourself hitting sticking points. This is a point past which you just can't seem to get any stronger, by either doing more reps and sets, adding more weight, or indeed moving onto a harder progression of a movement. In other words, you will hit plateaus in your performance, when it will seem impossible to overcome the barrier you have come up against. A barrier that is preventing you from improving any further.

This can be overcome with advanced techniques like cycling (which is covered in book 2 of this series, *Bodyweight Exercise: Exercise Programming,* in terms of programming specifically to keep making the best strength gains).

But this can also be overcome by remaining consistent in terms of the exercises you do, but by simply varying the approaches you use to each exercise. This will be especially true as you start progressing onto harder exercises which will require much more practice over a longer period of time to make even small amounts of progress.

These different approaches include the following:

- Dynamic approach
- Isometric approach
- Purposefully adjusting the range of motion from rep-to-rep to target particular portions of a given movement

With these different approaches you will vary how you perform the exercises you do so that you alter the time under tension that you subject your muscles to. Since tension equals force (7), and so strength where your muscles are concerned, the longer you place your muscles under tension for, the stronger you will become in these positions by forcing them to work at a greater level of effort or intensity.

Dynamic Approach

A dynamic approach just means working your muscles whilst moving, since your muscles will be contracting but whilst changing length. This will ideally occur by working through the whole range of motion of the movement, at a steady pace. This will target strengthening your muscles equally at each portion of the movement. But this will as such only strengthen these muscles in a limited manner since your muscles will only be kept under tension throughout the whole range of the motion for only a very brief amount of time.

To add time under tension with this approach, you can add intensity by simply slowing a phase of the movement down. An example would be counting for a set amount of time every time you lower into a movement, like the lowering portion of a pull-up or a push-up. (The lowering phase of any exercise is when the muscle lengthens, and is also called the eccentric phase).

To see how slowing down the eccentric phase of exercises can be effective, simply do ten push-ups at a normal, steady speed, both in terms of the lowering and rising (concentric phase), phases of the movement. Now, repeat your ten push-ups, but lower yourself for a count of 4 seconds, before coming back up at a normal speed, and see how much more strength this requires.

Isometric Approach

An isometric approach means that you will be contracting your muscles but that your muscles will remain the same length throughout the duration of the contraction. So in other words, you will lock your muscles in a set position and hold this position for time.

Using a ring push-up as an example exercise this time, since you can lower yourself much deeper than when doing push ups on the floor, an isometric approach could involve lowering yourself half way, before pausing and holding this position for 5 seconds with your elbows bent at 90 degrees. Then continue to the bottom position, and on your way back up, hold the 90 degree arm position again. Or do your push-ups as usual, but hold the bottom position for a prolonged period before coming back up.

This is a particularly effective way to get past a plateau in strength since you can very specifically target your weakest portion of a movement.

Why does this work?

Well, if you think about doing any exercise dynamically, your muscles are only actually passing through any part of the movement in a matter of a second or less. So if you are weak at any phase in a movement, by simply doing more repetitions, your muscles will still only get a limited amount of work in this weakest portion of the movement, and at a limited level of tension—say for a second for each repetition. So doing ten reps will only give you a total of a ten second contraction in this weakest position, and only very momentarily and at a comparatively weak level of tension since a moving muscle cannot contract as maximally as a stationery muscle. (If you don't believe this, just try to really tense your arm and move it as though to push an object away from you, as fast as you can. Importantly, keep the muscles as tense as possible. Now repeat the movement, but just move your arm in a normal, relaxed fashion and see how much faster you can move your arm. This demonstrates how the levels of tension vary greatly in relation to the speed at which you conduct a movement).

If you identify where you are weak in a movement though and hold this position for a full ten seconds, your muscles will remain tense in this particular portion of a movement for a continuous ten seconds. The resultant contraction will be at a very high intensity since you will have to tense your muscles much harder to lock yourself in position. This will force your muscles to get stronger in this particular phase of a movement much more effectively than by just doing more repetitions, since your muscles work at this higher level of tension for an extended, undisrupted period and so in a much more quality way.

This is also a simple method to integrate into your training, since if you need to target lots of phases of the movement in this way, you simply have to move into each position and hold as required.

To highlight the effectiveness of isometric exercises, particularly those that target your body as a whole within the movement, consider a plank. Many people will find this an extremely challenging exercise the first time of asking if you don't do planks frequently, or have never done one before. So this will immediately demonstrate how you have to really tense so many of your muscles just to hold this locked, static position.

As a result then, even such a seemingly simple movement can really strengthen your core in a manner that has lots of carry over to other movements. In particular, your push-ups will benefit, and also any movement that requires an understanding of holding your body straight and rigid. This is especially true as you progress onto working in a hollow position that requires only a slight alteration to your plank position. Yet this will have applicable carry over to so many advanced bodyweight and gymnastic type movements. Whether these movements are front levers, handstands, or planches, to name a few.

The plank will also demonstrate why bodyweight compound movements like push-ups are so effective as a form of training. Since you have to do a plank for the whole duration of your set of push-ups, albeit whilst your arms move rather than being locked, push-up movements develop core strength as well as the strength of the main muscles being targeted (the chest and triceps). A demonstration then of how a push-up—or any bodyweight movement reliant on this kind of position hold and the hollow hold—is really a total body exercise.

Adjusting the range of motion from rep-to-rep

In a similar way, targeting specific ranges of a movement in which you are weak, but integrated in amongst a dynamic movement, will add time under tension for your muscles during these weakest phases of your movements whilst still providing you with practice at the overall movement.

An example of this would be if you are weak in the top phase of a pull-up. If pulling from the start position seems okay, but getting your chin above the bar from about the half way up point is much harder than initiating the movement, specifically target this phase of the movement.

To do this, do 1 full pull-up rep. But then, as you come down, only lower halfway, to where your elbows are bent at 90 degrees. Hold this position for a few seconds or just momentarily at first. Next though, instead of lowering to the bottom hang, pull-up again from this 90 degree position so that your chin goes above the bar. Only then lower yourself all the way down to the bottom hang position before completing another full pull-up eccentric.

In this way, you are getting more practice, and very specifically practice at the top position that you may be weakest at by doing 1 full (up), 1 half (down, with the added benefit of an isometric hold), 1 half (up), 1 full (down) pull-up, and so on and so forth.

Or you could target the bottom position in the same way, by doing a full rep to the top with a full eccentric back to the bottom. Then on your next rep, only pull half way up and hold the 90 degree arm bend there for a few seconds, before lowering back down to pull-up into another full rep so that you focus more work on the initial pull position. This will again place your muscles under tension for a greater amount of time in the portion of the movement that is weakest for you, but still allow you to practice the full range of motion as well to ingrain this developing strength into the whole movement pattern.

So don't immediately take hitting a plateau in a specific exercise as a sign that you need to change the exercise that you are doing. Using any of the methods explained above, simply alter your approach to these exercises, so that you can again overcome these plateaus and so move past them and beyond by training smarter.

Summary

- From time-to-time you will hit plateaus in your training. This is where it seems like you just can't progress past a certain level of strength that you have achieved
- This is when you need to be smarter about your training by tricking your body into overcoming the plateau
- This does not mean you need to change the exercises that you do
- Instead, you just need to change your approach to the exercises that you already do to improve the effort or intensity of these movements to gain the strength to overcome the plateau
- Or you can apply periodisation in a strength targeted way

Principle 10
The Importance of Strength
Train specifically for strength from time to time to build more size

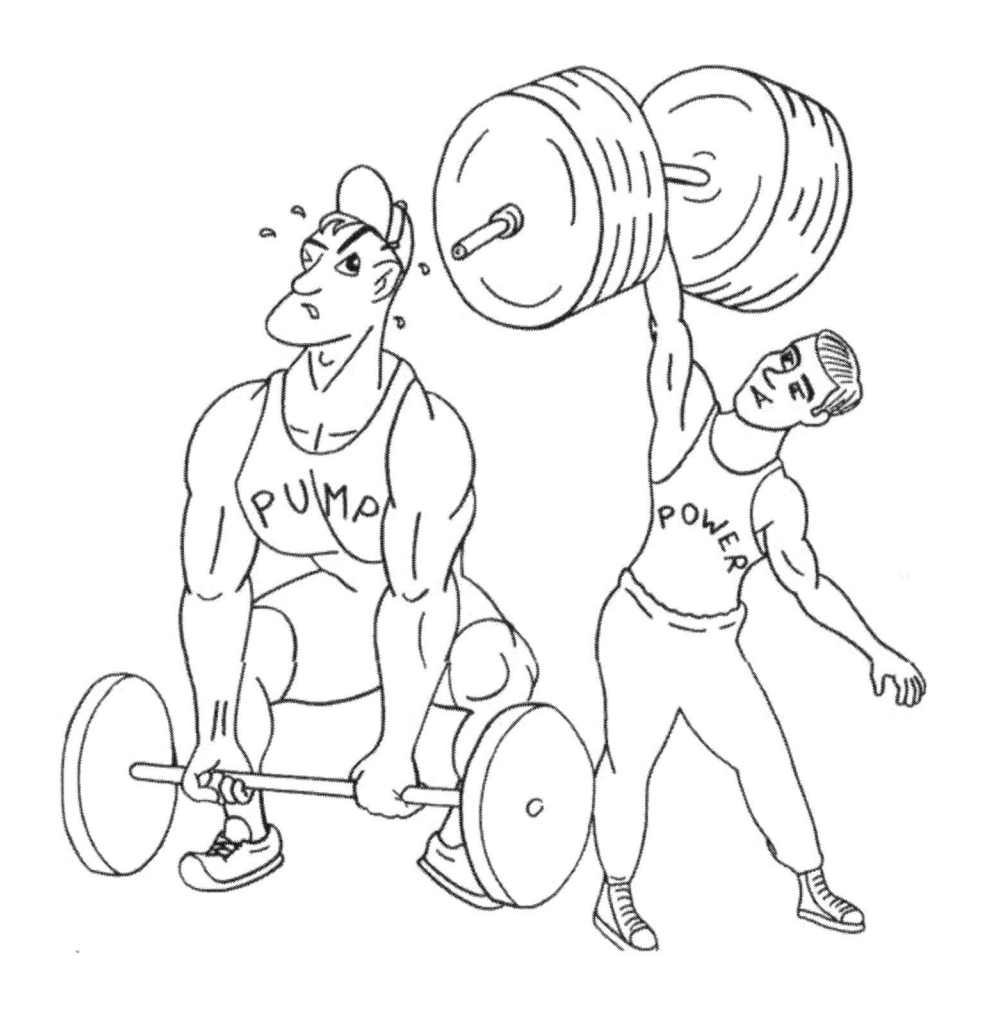

"No citizen has a right to be an amateur in the matter of physical training … What a disgrace it is for a man to grow old without ever seeing the beauty and strength of which his body is capable."

Socrates

This principle may seem really obvious. Of course you have to get stronger to get bigger in terms of growing larger muscles.

But as highlighted at the beginning of this book, building maximum strength will allow you to improve both muscular growth and muscular endurance.

If you have read anything about exercising to build muscle, you will surely have come across the idea of training in different set and rep ranges in order to get different results from training. Here is how this will help you to adjust your training in terms of reps and sets from time-to-time so that you can specifically target improving maximal strength, growth, or muscular endurance.

This can easily and quickly be summed up in a table relating to reps as below:

Strength Range	Hypertrophy Range	Endurance Range
1 – 5 reps	8 - 15 reps	15 reps and above

There is some leeway on this, and this is a generalisation, but this is generally what has been found to work best in terms of developing these various attributes.

So, when I say you should train for strength to build more size, I specifically mean that in order to get bigger, you need to be able to lift greater loads or to do harder progressions of bodyweight exercises so that you are handling greater loads over time. This will ensure that you are working at a progressively higher intensity as time goes on so that you keep getting results from your training.

When put in practice, this means that you need to ensure that once an exercise has become too easy, you again increase the difficulty and so intensity.

In practical terms, this 'easy' point is where you are able to do 15 repetitions (or up to 20 repetitions to be on the safe side with bodyweight movements and create a comfort zone), for sets on a given version of an exercise. Any more repetitions than this, and you are working on improving muscular endurance only, which is no good for developing your muscle in terms of size. So if you are looking to build size, then to keep getting bigger, you need to move onto a harder version of an exercise, or add more weight to that movement so that you are again working to develop strength so that you can again move back into the hypertrophy rep range with time.

If using weights of course, you could just increase the weight you use in the same exercise, and so work on this in the 8-15 rep range again. Or, with bodyweight exercises, you can also add weight in some way, and do the same, such as by using a dipping belt to add weights to your dips.

However, when you jump a progression in your bodyweight exercises, such as from feet elevated rows to tuck front lever rows, you will again encounter a much greater need for strength just by having altered the version of the exercise you are doing.

So, to ensure that this new version of the exercise is hard enough, choose an exercise variant or a weight that you use in that exercise that allows you to do five repetitions. If you feel you could maybe do one or two more reps, that is fine too, but initially, just focus on doing sets of five in that exercise and adding sets until you can do 5 reps for 3-5 sets. Only once you can do 3-5 sets x 5 reps comfortably, and you have ideally been doing this set and rep pattern for six weeks, should you again start working on doing more reps in any of your sets so that you move into the 8-15 rep range again.

Since maximal strength is best trained by low reps but high intensity, if you really want to focus on developing greater strength alone without building any muscle mass, as some sports like climbing and gymnastics require however, stick to sets of 5 reps for lower sets, so 2 to 3 sets maximum. In general, where max strength is concerned, less is more, especially for the reasons of best recovery and so the ability to exercise with a higher frequency. (Frequency being important to strength since, as shown in Principles 2 and 5, strength development requires neurological adaptations and so skill development, and skills require regular practice).

By doing either of these low rep approaches then, you will really have to focus on the form, but also will be working on developing brute strength before any other attribute by expressly developing your nervous system and fast twitch muscle fibres again. This will in time build your strength for the reasons already mentioned and allow you to start building up to doing more repetitions of the same exercise with correct form, since you are now strong enough to do that movement comfortably for more reps.

Not only will this build the foundational strength that you require in a new, harder move then, improving the safety of your workouts, but you can also use this rep and set scheme as a useful way to measure your increasing strength. So your rep ranges can be used as an intensity monitor. After all, the ability to do only 5 reps of a move is a simple way to tell you that you are again working at the correct intensity from which to start making strength improvements again at the correct level for you. So this will inform your trial and error when it comes to setting your training at your correct level, thus helping to inform your goal setting.

Summary

- Building high levels of maximum strength is the foundation that will lead to you being able to build muscle and muscular endurance in harder bodyweight progressions, or with higher weights in weighted exercises
- When working on elevating your level of strength alone, on occasion, focus on trying to achieve 3-5 sets of 5 reps of an exercise. Ideally, repeat this 3-5 x 5 rep pattern for at least six weeks so that your neurological adaptations will have chance to occur, or longer as required
- Only once this strength foundation has been laid down for the new progression should you start increasing the number of reps you perform back to the 8-15 rep range that will better target muscular growth

Conclusion

Here you have them then. 10 principles that if employed and applied to your workouts will be sure to give you the best results and on an ongoing basis.

As you will have seen, many of these principles relate to forcing you to apply higher levels of effort through various techniques. These include practicing correct form, mindful training, and utilising different training approaches to help overcome plateaus to build higher levels of strength. This really is key as time progresses in order to keep forcing yourself to get results, and to prevent your progress from stagnating.

These principles really are the basics of how to get an exercise program to work, but all too often these seemingly obvious things can be missed, and often the cause of not getting the results you might expect lies somewhere in these simple but fundamental principles.

So if at any time you stop getting the results from your workouts that you desire for a prolonged period of time, or you are currently failing to get any results, don't just keep plugging away at your workouts in the hope that you will get a different outcome at some point.

Instead, learn to stand back and critically assess what you might be doing wrong. For this purpose, use this list of principles as a checklist if you will, and question if you are applying each of these principles in some way in your workouts. If you are, this may just be a matter of employing more time to push through the plateau, but if you aren't, identify which of these principles is lacking from your training, and adjust your training accordingly.

References

(1) Shima N, Ishida, K.Katayama, K.Morotome, Y.Sato,Y.Miyamura, M. Cross education of muscular strength during unilateral resistance training and detraining. Eur J Appl Physiol 2002; 86: 287-294

(2) Paavolainen L, Paavolainen L, Hakkinen K, et al. Explosive-strength training improves 5-km running time by improving running economy and muscle power. J Appl Physiol 1999; 86: 1527-1533

(3) Kongsgaard M, Aagaard P, Kjaer M, et al. Structural Achilles tendon properties in athletes subjected to different exercise modes and in Achilles tendon rupture patients. J Appl Physiol 2005 in press;

(4) Schoenfeld, Brad J (2010), 'The Mechanisms of Muscle Hypertrophy and Their Application to Resistance Training' [online] http://www.lookgreatnaked.com/articles/mechanisms_of_muscle_hypertrophy.pdf (Accessed 20/02/2017).

(5) Ralston, Peter (2006), *Zen Body Being: An Enlightened Approach to Physical Skill, Grace, and Power*, California, Frog Ltd.

(6) Alway SE, Grumbt WH, Stray-Gundersen J, et al. Effects of resistance training on elbow flexors of highly competitive bodybuilders. J Appl Physiol 1992; 72: 1512-21

(7) Tsatsouline, Pavel (2000), *Power to the People,* United States, Dragon Door Publications, Inc.

Appendix 1
Why building max strength will also help to build endurance

Muscle tissue, in the form of the individual muscle cells, are where your metabolism, or the production of energy in your body, takes place, and this energy is produced by a process called respiration. To state it simply, metabolism is just the process by which your body releases energy from the food that you eat to produce energy and also growth, so includes all the chemical reactions that contribute towards this.

At the beginning of this book, I touched on the idea that muscles are responsible for two kinds of strength:

1. Maximum strength
2. Strength endurance

There is often a misconception that cardio exercise is separate from your muscles however. In other words, exercises considered to be cardio workouts like jogging, cycling, or any prolonged, but low intensity activity, like walking even, which build endurance, are considered as cardio workouts.

The cardio or cardiovascular system, however, consists of your heart, lungs, and circulatory system. And this is inextricably linked to your muscles since it is this cardiovascular apparatus that delivers oxygen to your muscles which is where the actual metabolism takes place.

Importantly though, metabolism, and more specifically the respiration reactions can, occur either in the presence of oxygen, or when oxygen is absent. This is called aerobic and anaerobic respiration respectively. When you work at a low intensity, the aerobic metabolic pathways produce most of your energy, and when you work very hard, but for shorter periods of time, your anaerobic metabolic pathways are used.

Consequently, whilst resistance workouts like weights or calisthenics, (bodyweight resistance training), may be looked upon as strength workouts with little cardiovascular benefit, this is a wrong way to look at exercise, since all exercise works your metabolism and is, as such, cardiovascular exercise.

Furthermore however, resistance workouts are, very importantly, higher in intensity or effort than prolonged, but low intensity exercise considered to be endurance targeting workouts, like jogging. And where exercise is concerned, intensity is everything.

Because of how metabolism in muscle cells works, energy enters your muscle cells and passes along anaerobic pathways before reaching the aerobic apparatus of the cell: the mitochondria. And really taxing the anaerobic energy systems in the cell produces more energy more quickly than the aerobic energy system can.

Importantly however, exercise performed at high intensity causes a number of important things to happen to your metabolism:

- Drains the glycogen stores held in your muscle cells
- Triggers the use of fat stored in your body's fat cells already, so, in other words, burns fat, which is then also used to produce energy
- Produces waste products like lactic acid. The removal of these occurs in the days after you have worked out via aerobic metabolism so that your aerobic metabolism works at the same rate, or greater, than it would do if you were jogging or walking for a prolonged time. This afterburner effect, if you want to call it that, is known as EPOC (Exercise Post Oxygen Consumption)
- Builds more muscle, which in future will amplify all of the above effects on an ongoing basis
- Teaches your body to better absorb oxygen into the muscle tissues by causing adaptations to your blood cells to this end. So your muscular endurance will actually improve since your heart won't have to work as hard to get the same amounts of oxygen to your tissues

For these reasons then, resistance workouts will actually do many of the things more usually associated with 'cardio workouts,' and many things they cannot do for your health. This is why resistance workouts should absolutely be a part of any workout program aimed at causing weight loss.

Be sure to review this book

If any of the information in this book helped you at all, in any way, please be sure to leave a review for this book on the Amazon page where you purchased it. It is my goal to help as many people as possible in their quest for a higher level of fitness, and your reviews will help my material reach the greatest number of people.

Also, this book is the first in a series of books I will be writing so keep your eyes peeled for more to come.

The next book, *Bodyweight Exercise: Exercise Programming*, will be available soon from my website, www.trainyourselffit.com, and Amazon.

In this next book in the series you will learn how to:

- Put all of the principles learnt in this book into practice when designing your own workout programs
- Everything you'll need to design your own, tailor made work outs, to specifically target the results you want, whether this is to grow bigger muscles, to get stronger without gaining any muscle, or just to get the best all round results for overall body development
- What to consider and so how to select the exercises you choose to do in your workout programs
- How to ensure you work at the right levels of intensity in your workouts to ensure you keep getting long term benefits from exercise i.e. throughout your life
- How to guarantee you will keep making progress in your training by incorporating progressive overload into your training at the right times, and how to identify when to do this
- How to structure your workout programs week-to-week and longer term using periodisation
- How to use periodisation as a powerful tool to keep getting results from your workouts when many others often just stagnate and plateau
- Various examples of different ways to structure your workout programs to get results

You can also visit my website for online training to get one-to-one coaching from me, and to read my fitness blog, at www.trainyourselffit.com.

Thank you for reading and good luck with your training.

Printed in Great Britain
by Amazon